KU-250-547

The Black Lace Book of
Women's Sexual Fantasies

The Black Lace Book of Women's Sexual Fantasies

COMPILED AND EDITED BY
KERRI SHARP

Black Lace books contain sexual fantasies.
In real life, make sure you practise safe sex.

First published in 1999 by
Black Lace
Thames Wharf Studios,
Rainville Road, London W6 9HT

Reprinted 1999, 2000

Copyright © Virgin Publishing Ltd and Kerri Sharp
1999

Typeset by SetSystems Ltd, Saffron Walden, Essex
Printed and bound by Mackays of Chatham PLC

ISBN 0 352 33346 4

This book is sold subject to the condition that it shall
not, by way of trade or otherwise, be lent, resold, hired
out or otherwise circulated without the publisher's
prior written consent in any form of binding or cover
other than that in which it is published and without a
similar condition including this condition being
imposed on the subsequent purchaser.

Contents

*To hedonists and rebels everywhere;
and to the nuns of St Joseph's Convent for
making me a hedonist and rebel for life.*

Chapter One

A Personal History: Good Girls, Bad Girls and Why Fantasies Matter

When I was seventeen years old, a woman called Ruth lent me her copy of Nancy Friday's *My Secret Garden*. I had never read anything like it, and it would be fair to say that the book changed my life. It made me realise I was not alone; I was not the freak I thought I was. It affirmed something I had long suspected but had been unsure of discussing – that women had elaborate sexual fantasies that were not always about romance and that were sometimes shocking and 'not nice'. I saw the book as a vindication of my rights, although I didn't express my feelings in such confident terms at the time. I kept the book close to my person and, through lowered eyes, shyly told my boyfriend of the time, 'It's quite interesting, actually.' In fact it was like having a time bomb in my hands, so exciting and empowering was the stuff I was reading. I still have that same copy of the book. I never did give it back to Ruth. If she's out there somewhere, I want to say thanks – that was the best present anyone

1

could have given me at that time. It was my first adult encounter with explicit material written by and for women. Its influence lasted: fifteen years later I would be involved in the creation of a list of fiction which shaped a new genre and turned female fantasies into novels.

I grew up aware that sexuality was channelled through images of women. To my young eyes, to be 'sexy' was synonymous with being female; images of men held no fascination for me, but I would gaze for hours at pictures of beauty queens: Miss Worlds, Bond girls and high-fashion models of the 1970s. I knew that sexy women had Factor X, and that men wanted it. I thought an exciting world of adult fun lay ahead of me. I didn't want my future relationships with men to be a copy of the drudgery the women of my mother's generation seemed to endure. I was aware that my life would be different. I would take control of my desires, explore all the possibilities of a modern life. I would have fun! What I found when I was old enough to have fun, though, was a narrow-minded view as to which kinds of sexuality were acceptable. It was OK to be a sexy woman with Factor X as long as you were physically stunning and, above all else, had an unthreatening personality; your sexiness had to be palatable to men. If it didn't conform to their ideal – or if you were unsure whether you were gay or straight – it was best that you kept your sexuality to yourself.

Like many young teens, I'd accidentally stumbled across porn mags but, because they didn't cater to a female audience, there seemed to be little about them that was empowering or entertaining. After the initial reaction of giggling at something naughty had subsided, I began to feel cheated: it was as if my gender wasn't being allowed to share in that exciting world of adult fun. The only voice being heard was the male voice; the only erotic images being displayed were the images men had chosen. As women, we were the ones who were there to be looked at, the ones who took the passive role. 'Men look at women. Women watch themselves being looked at,' writes John Berger in *Ways of Seeing*.[1] The idea of being the gender that did the looking, or of producing explicit material for a female audience, was revolutionary, and had to wait some fifteen years before coming into being. Moralists and feminists told us that women didn't want such a product; it was off limits. We would have to be happy with our romantic novels and dreams of ideal homes.

I thought it unfair – and a sweeping generalisation – to be told that we didn't like or want material that was sexually explicit. This notion seemed far more sexist than the pornography we were being told was the big bad wolf. There was little cultural evidence around at the time to support my belief, and this is why Nancy Friday's book was such a revelation. In the working-class milieu in which I grew up, single girls who liked sex were 'slags', and, if you were to embark on a journey of sexual discovery, you would pay for it with your reputation. Words such as 'holistic' and 'empowering' weren't in the general vocabulary of East London in the mid-70s, and to be open about your sexuality was to invite ridicule and disrespect from boys and scornful finger-wagging from feminist friends.

I was confused. I was a strong-willed young woman who wanted equal opportunities; I knew where I stood politically. But I was being told by the people I admired that my sex drive was a false consciousness, my desires were misguided and that I had been brainwashed by men. I didn't want to contradict these people as they were the ones fighting for equal opportunities at work and taking steps to combat racism. I felt trapped in a paradox. It was drummed into me that a young woman couldn't pursue an active sex life

3

without being exploited. At the same time I was adamant that my desires were nobody else's business. I felt sure there was a way around this but, until I found what that route was, I was going to investigate as many alternative lifestyles as possible and investigate some of the history of sexual thinking.

Reading *My Secret Garden* had created in me a fascination for explicit material in text form. I wanted to see what else was out there. I sought out the works of Anaïs Nin, Colette and Erica Jong. Like many of the women who contributed fantasies to this book, I read *The Story of O* by Pauline Réage. I learnt about SM practices, and how the theatricality necessary for their performance was a way of having sex on a different, more elaborate and somehow more artistic level. I was steered in the direction of literary erotica; to the works of Georges Bataille and the surrealists; I was fascinated by the art of the Pre-Raphaelites and the *fin de siècle* hedonism of Beardsley and the decadent aesthetes. I believed there was more to sex than snogging boys at the disco or having an unsatisfactory fumble on the sofa. I was interested in the part imagination had to play in sexuality. I thought there should be something of artistic merit in this whole business; something cathartic, liberating and almost religious. In my personal life I kept coming up against men's shock, resistance and disbelief. One thing became clear: women with a strong sexuality were threatening to men.

At the age of seventeen I was studying art history at college, and much of the discourse was taken up with analysing that ever-popular subject of European art: the nude woman. She was nearly always passive; laid bare for man's pleasure, her gaze directed at the viewer, awaiting his approval. The similarities between the high art of figurative oil painting and the 'lowbrow' mass culture of pornography for men were obvious. However, as John Berger points out, 'It is worth notic-

4

ing that in non-European traditions – in Indian, Persian, African and Pre-Columbian art ... when the theme of a work is sexual attraction, it is likely to show active sexual love between two people, the woman as active as the man, the actions of each absorbing the other.'[2] There was nothing to parallel this interpretation in the art of the Judeo-Christian world, and I couldn't find any pornography that showed men and women enjoying *each other's* bodies.

Western art has consistently portrayed the sexual woman as slothful, indulgent, vain and fickle; the antithesis of all that is godly, good or wholesome. Throughout the history of the past two thousand years, women have been encouraged (through varying degrees of force) to present a face of modesty. Our sexualities are treated with fear or suspicion unless they conform to rules of good behaviour. Our desires will be tolerated only if they are perceived as 'safe' and unthreatening, forever wrapped up in notions of romance, love and nurturing. A more voracious female sexuality is seen as an aberration and likely to transform into an anarchic force if it is given free rein. 'It seems absurd,' as the artist Lydia Lunch points out in *Suture*, 'that we live in a society where it's legitimate to use a woman's sexuality to sell everything, but she can't sell her own body, or even use it in the way she wants to.'[3]

Western society's relationship with the sexual woman has a history of being rooted in hypocrisy. Take, for example, the women in the US film noir of the 1940s and 50s: the female characters who have chosen not to conform to the ideal of being a caring wife or mother are the bad girls, the ones who will wreck the home and steal your husbands and get involved in larceny and murder. But they are also the most magnetic; the ones who demand our attention and who are the most desirable. In the mainstream

5

Hollywood narrative, this type of female character almost without exception meets a grisly end, unless, of course, she renounces her sins and becomes a born-again good girl. To me, bad girls are far more interesting as characters. Their refusal to conform, their defiance of patriarchal finger-wagging, their love of late nights, of dancing, flashy clothes and fast cars, make far more attractive role models than the dutiful servants and loyal wives who find fulfilment only in servicing the needs of others.

In the latter half of the 1970s, it seemed the dominant message to women via mass culture hadn't changed that much from the seventeenth-century painting or the film noir. We were still being told to behave ourselves and conform if we wanted respect and an easy life. Luckily, the punk scene exploded in London in 1977 and began to shake things up a bit. Being an *enfant terrible* became synonymous with producing interesting new forms of art, music and literature. Breaking the rules and upsetting the conformists became fun; shock and outrage were good reactions to what the kids were doing. It was a time of unparalleled expression of defiance. Across the country, young people were turning their rebellion into an art form. Anger was an energy and life was very exciting.

This was the way round the paradox, then: making the personal political and looking behind the arguments about decency and morality to find the real agenda for censoring and negating half the world's sexuality. I was keen to find out what was the collective experience of other young women. I remember asking my friends and contemporaries about their experience of sex – what had they learnt and been told? Were they happy with the dominant cultural representation of their gender's aspirations and sexual ambitions? Mostly, the answers were a sad indictment of the state many young people's relationships were in. Young women were afraid to tell their boyfriends what they really wanted in bed because they didn't want to be thought of as 'cheap' or 'sluttish'. At that time it was still unusual for women to admit to reading explicit material. Writing about sex for women was largely a medical issue, confined to the pages of women's magazines, whose focus was on fashion and beauty and not autonomous sexual enjoyment.

Attitudes did change a little, however, and the feisty women of punk music, women such as Siouxsie Sioux of Siouxsie and the Banshees and Poly Styrene of X-Ray Spex, gave young women alternative role models who were spiky, talented and had strong opinions. This was the first time that pop culture had given us women who created themselves in their own image; women who wouldn't stand for being told to look conventially pretty and sing 'nice' songs. A few years later, female sexuality became closely linked to the 80s obsessions with power and success. Capitalism reappropriated the strong woman for itself. To have an active, satisfying or risqué sex life, you had to be like Joan Collins' character Alexis, in *Dynasty* – in other words, privileged. We could escape into a world of glitz, where lovers were desired, devoured and spat out, and where women were glamorous and exciting. At least we could now vicariously enjoy an adventurous sex life even if our day-to-day reality was located in the supermarket and the office, rather than country clubs, glittering parties and Texan boardrooms. The woman's blockbuster novels – such as those by Jilly Cooper and Jackie Collins – established themselves as the place where 'women's issues' were tackled through narrative; they found a huge audience. Feminist discourse was worthy and necessary, but it seemed to have a puritanical face to women who wanted a bit of escapism. Books such as *Lace* by Shirley Conran offered what Avis Lewallen called 'a mini-encyclopaedia of female sexuality', dealing as they do with 'loss of virginity, sexual desire, sexual satisfaction and frigidity, to prostitution, rape, adultery, lesbianism, and transvestism. [It] also deals with pornography, alcoholism, plastic surgery, childbirth, miscarriage, and abortion.'[4] Lewallen entitled her essay *'Lace: Pornography for Women?'* although the pejorative tone implicit in the word 'pornography' was more a reference to the suspicion with which many feminist writers viewed the women's novel than her own analysis of the genre. She concluded her essay with the point that, through novels such as *Lace*, feminism managed a small but valuable intervention into the mass market, for the simple reason that women were portrayed as striving for their own financial independence: 'Men and sex and love [were] important to the female characters, but money – their own money – [was] more important'.[5] It would be interesting to see what Lewallen thinks about Black Lace books – the 90s successor to the women's 'bonkbuster' – where independence is a given and sex is the driving force of the narrative.

Society was about to be shocked into reality in the early 80s when a sexual issue began to dominate the headlines. Everyone was made to sit up and take notice, regardless of social status. The slogan was 'Don't Die of Ignorance'; the issue was AIDS. It would force us into discussing previously taboo subjects in the public arena. If one good thing came about from the panic surrounding how the virus was contracted, it was surely the emergence of a new realism about sexual behaviour. Apart from the tiny but vociferous minority who wanted to use the tragedy as a soapbox on which to drone on about family values and punishment from God, most people recognised the need to face up to the facts: young people had lots of sex – some had lots of partners – and failure to address the consequences of unprotected intercourse could prove fatal. A new awareness began to appear: sales of condoms multiplied, lovers began to talk to each other and safe sex was the only sex to be having if you didn't have a regular partner. Safe sex became groovy: condoms were suddenly fruity and colourful and available in both men's and women's toilets. Also, the emerging loved-up dance culture of the late 1980s pushed the focus further towards sensuality and non-penetrative love play. People were learning to be more creative during sex, and communicating with your partner was not as embarrassing as it had been in previous decades.

The 90s has seen a period of greater tolerance emerge; we are less easily shocked but more cynical about sex. However, it's not a good idea to get too complacent. In reality there may be a relaxation by people at a grass-roots level towards explicit material, but in many places this new climate has yet to be reflected by changes to the law. While informed, media-literate people in London and San Francisco debate sexuality in terms of self-expression and fashion, in law – at least in the UK – the definition of what is obscene is as clear as mud and is rooted in Victorian ideas of what is liable to deprave and corrupt. As we approach the twenty-first century, many politicians and moral crusaders are still having a problem dragging themselves out of the nineteenth. The pro-censorship lobby seems unable to accept that humans have a fantasy life that is liberating, pleasurable and harmless, and that is just one facet of the multifaceted beings we are. Being sexual is one of the many things we can be; we don't have to sacrifice our rights as women, employees, citizens or consumers because we sometimes like to allow our imaginations free rein.

It is easy for those who have a vested interest – or religious or political reasons – in censoring free speech to whip up hysteria over material which is sexually

9

explicit. I must stress that by this I mean material that is produced by adults, featuring adults, for adults. When the media reports that customs has seized a shipment of 'hardcore pornography', this deliberately plays on the fears of ordinary people and conjures up worst-case scenarios of snuff movies, violence and brutal imagery that no healthy person would get off on. In fact, 'hardcore' is an umbrella term for images that feature erections and penetrative intercourse; images not that different from the non-European art of previous centuries: the *Kama Sutra*, the pottery of Ancient Greece, the Pillow Books of Japan. Perhaps there may be some oral sex, too, or shots of male ejaculation. Maybe the models are enjoying themselves too much; setting a bad example. I doubt, however, that British society will descend into anarchy because the penis is on display. Why does Britain have such a problem with the human male erection?

Recently, at the Erotica exhibition at London's Olympia, colour portrait photographs – very much in the 'art' vein – of men with full erections had stickers slapped over the 'offending' parts by the Vice Squad. Other photographs featuring the semi-hard penis were allowed. Twenty degrees makes all the difference when you run the risk of prosecution. The exhibition was open only to persons over eighteen years of age and the subject of the images were definitely adults. Now, as has always been the case, censors lack sophistication in that they are alarmist, reactionary and, more often than not, uneducated in the history of art; and visual irony escapes them completely.

No genre has had to defend itself as vigorously against accusation as erotica, and erotica produced by women is viewed with most suspicion of all. It is always guilty until proven innocent. We have to justify every nuance, every storyline, every fantasy, because we're constantly reminded that pornography is for men only, and women shouldn't want it. If we are allowed to have some, then it has to be somehow 'nicer' than what men like because, after all, we are women, and women are the guardians, the mothers, the teachers, the vulnerable, and the protectors of all that is vulnerable. We cannot be seen to be actively sexual and concerned with self-indulgence. We should be caring and nurturing, and not contributing to moral anarchy by flaunting our sexuality.

What is particularly depressing is hearing patriarchal dogma coming from the mouths of young people; disadvantaged young men, mostly, who seem unable to realise that these outdated misogynist concepts of good girls and whores don't benefit anyone. The greatest way to defeat our disadvantages is to recognise who wields the power in our society and stop making moral judgements about people who make up our own peer group, whether we're black, white, unemployed, working too hard, under stress or undervalued. Moral panic is a distraction. Our planet is blighted by poverty, war, genocide, prejudice and pollution – things far more destructive and damaging than sexually explicit material, be it videos, magazines, books or strip shows. I would challenge anyone to convince me that women have a better time in countries where pornography is banned. The happiest and kindest people I meet tend to be those who are tolerant. The inevitable consequence of intolerance is political extremism, which benefits no one except a few self-appointed dictators and their lackeys. This may sound alarmist, but we don't have to look very far into history to see what happens when book-burning and censorship gets out of hand.

Over the course of the past five years – since Black Lace books have been around – I and some of my authors have regularly been asked to appear on television. Usually it's the same old chestnut of a question:

11

do women really want to read pornography? When I answer that yes, *some* women *sometimes* want to read explicit material, the stern-faced opponents are ready to point accusatory fingers at me; to tell me that feminists have fought for years for women's equality, for fair practice in the workplace, for changes in the law that benefit women and so on, and that by producing books such as Black Lace I am in some way letting the side down. No other series of books has been accused of 'corrupting the morals of the nation's women and betraying civilised values', as one Sunday tabloid newspaper put it in 1993. These words still make me smile. Far from uniting the country against the 'degrading filth', reactionary articles such as this ensured that the first four titles went into seven reprints apiece. Authors can write crime fiction, murder mysteries, horror, science fiction or romance but never are they made to justify the existence of their chosen area of interest – and nor should they be expected to. It is fantasy. It is fiction. The works are novels. Going against the prescriptive formula that says we are meant to find fulfilment only in servicing the needs of others makes us the bad girls. My authors are guilty of the sin of indulgence and I am guilty of paying for the fruits of that indulgence. As Avedon Carol notes in *Bad Girls and Dirty Pictures*, 'By choosing to write or read explicit material, or to seek our own pleasure, we're guilty of committing that greatest of female sins: selfishness.'[6]

She continues, 'Sex for pleasure is treated as a male vice, and women who like sex and are expressive about their sexuality are seen as victims of male propaganda. If we admit to taking pleasure from sexuality expressed outside of a "loving, equal relationship", or in unconventional acts, we are seen to be legitimising male violence rather than acting assertively.'[7] In the UK, female sexuality is still treated with either suspicion or derision. Back in 1973, Nancy Friday was accused of making up the fantasies in *My Secret Garden*. Twenty years later many journalists thought Black Lace books were written by men using pseudonyms. The late 1990s has seen a proliferation of features in women's magazines concerned with 'great sex and how to get it', but those glossy pages show us a very sanitised variety of our sex lives. The accent is firmly fixed on fashion. The message says it's all right to have lots of good sex – but it'll be so much better if you're wearing designer clothes. Nice if you have the cash. It's important to remember that the escapism of sexual fantasy is available to us all, and need not be governed by the predetermined values of a culture that rewards only the privileged or conventionally beautiful. This is why collections of real women's fantasies are important. From the Nancy Friday books to this Black Lace collection, they validate the diversity of the imaginary experience and remind us that difference is good.

The book is divided into themed sections. Certain fantasies are notable for individuality or bizarreness. However, most fall into one of twelve categories by nature of the predominant element. Of course, some fantasies include a mixture of two or more elements. For instance, someone who is into thinking about group sex may well involve bondage or fetish clothes in their favourite scenario. It is impossible to draw absolute boundaries around a subject as multifaceted as the sexual imagination. However, I've tried as far as possible to categorise according to what I believe is the dominant element in each fantasy. All names have been changed to protect anonymity.

A significant number of the readers who sent back their questionnaires expressed their reticence to confess their fantasies to their men. This is either because they want to keep their fantasies as their own personal means of escape or they were worried the men would be scared off or not treat the information as confidential. When you grant someone anonymity, you are more likely to get their real opinion – the private opinion. The term 'public opinion' is usually applied to evidence that purports to be truth, but the paradox is that a private opinion is much more likely to be accurate.

If you are attached to a man, I hope you are lucky enough to have a boyfriend, lover or husband who realises he is blessed to have a partner who is open-minded and at ease with her sexuality. To be able to trust another person with your innermost thoughts is liberating and exciting. The sexiest thing a man can do for a woman is listen to her fantasies, remember what turns her on, and not be judgemental. Women are just beginning to be allowed sexual autonomy. The emergence of women-only sex shops such as SH! in the UK and Good Vibrations in the US are an essential alternative to retail outlets that have traditionally catered exclusively to men. Sex shops – in the UK at least – have always seemed seedy, unwelcoming and off limits to females. Often shabby and shy on decor, the atmosphere in such shops has done nothing to encourage openness or a sense of fun around the whole business.

Again, things are changing. Events such as the Erotica exhibition and numerous clubs where being sexy goes hand in hand with dressing up and having a good time mean that many people are beginning to recognise that sex as entertainment is a human interest. It is nothing to be ashamed of, and the idea that it should be restricted to one gender is absurd. Women are also becoming more involved in the production side of things. I hesitate to call it the sex industry; rather I think of it as one aspect of the entertainment business. As society becomes more sophisticated, more visually literate, we expect better products in all areas. Who would have thought, fifteen years ago, that you would be able to choose from a staggering amount of conveniently packaged foreign meals and twenty different types of olive in the local supermarket?

What this illustrates is that we are becoming used to having a huge amount of choice when it comes to spending our money. This choice should be allowed to extend to the adult market, too. The obscenity laws need to keep pace with cultural change. The antiquated notion that printed material or film is liable to 'deprave and corrupt' is a nonsense in a society where access to any information is available via the Internet. Until the day when rationality replaces alarmism around this issue, we shall continue to play those X-rated images in our minds. No legislation can probe into our imaginations, and the thought police of Orwellian dystopia shall, thankfully, remain a fantasy that will never come true.

I'd like to say a big thank you to every woman who contributed her fantasy to this project. The response was enormous, and I regret that it hasn't been possible to include everything in a book of this size. The human spirit is prey to the most astounding impulses and the human sexual imagination is diverse, sometimes shocking, fascinating, unpredictable and valid. I hope that this collection of our readers' fantasies illustrates that diversity.

Chapter Two

Stranger Attractions: Anonymity Guaranteed

Whatever your sexuality, I'm sure that you will have felt at some point an instant and powerful sexual attraction to a stranger. If that person caught you looking at him or her and returned your gaze, possibly adding an obvious sexual come-on signal, I bet a bolt of illicit pleasure went through you that you couldn't shake off for some time. It's nice when that happens; it affirms our desirability. But do we ever do anything about it? Only the very brave or drunken few. Unfortunately, we usually meet these people when we're changing trains on our way to work, or passing along the aisles in the supermarket; situations where we cannot easily strike up a conversation. We can never be sure that the person in question really did return our appreciative glance, so we're not going to run the risk of approaching them and stuttering out some pathetic introduction.

It's ironic that we can attend a hundred parties and not see one person who ignites the sexual spark we feel for that attractive stranger. The simplicity of what Erica Jong called the 'zipless fuck' makes instant sex very attractive. It's what animals do. To not get to know a person before sharing an act of ultimate intimacy goes against all our conditioning as caring human beings. For women, this is especially true. In reality – for a number of reasons – we pass these opportunities by rather than risk looking stupid or reckless. In our fantasies, however, we swallow our fear and go for it. We don't have to bother with condoms; we don't have to have the embarrassing silence afterwards ('Er, what was your name, by the way?'); and we don't have to continue our journey in a dishevelled state.

Many erotic stories are based on the traditional 'stranger on a train' theme. There's something very British about the idea of nipping off for a quick one with our object of desire in the train loo, and giggling like loons afterwards at the irate people who were queuing outside. A few drinks in the buffet car, loosened inhibitions because it's the weekend, and that rolling movement of the carriages seem to inspire people to do naughty things. It's the same principle at work that created the now clichéd idea of the mile-high club. It didn't surprise me that a number of fantasies arrived from our readers featuring trains, and for this reason I have decided to group them all together, even though Lisa's fantasy has elements of exhibitionism in it, and Chris's fantasy would certainly classify as group sex. However, it is the anonymity of the situation that provides the basis for the fantasy.

There's an element of danger to many of the anonymous fantasies, not least the prospect of being caught. The London listings magazine *Time Out* recently ran a survey of Londoners' sex habits, and found that twenty six per cent of their respondees had had sex in a public toilet, while twenty one per cent had done the nasty on public transport! Sex on an aeroplane scored only a measly five per cent, being beaten by seven per cent who claimed they'd got down to it in a cemetery.[1] While it's not possible to find out how many of those adventurous lovers were strangers to each other, the fantasies which follow are more likely to feature spontaneous sex, as we're not going to meet that attractive stranger in our homes.

There's a lot of downright dirty dialogue going on in these fantasies, especially in Janine's. I think it's symptomatic of the fact that we know we can let go because we are with a stranger; we don't have to worry about being thought of as 'easy', or that we have to look gorgeous because we're concerned with our loved one's pleasure. The sexy-stranger fantasy is about being able to be selfish for once. This is an indication of our imaginations working in subtle ways to relieve us of the guilt surrounding sex. It is sometimes difficult to be as liberated as we would like with our regular partner because so much trust is required and we've made so much emotional investment. This is the reason why cyberspace has become such a popular place to conduct X-rated chat. We can assume a different sex and identity without fear of discovery. It's the ultimate anonymous experience and the ultimate safe sex.

Terri, 26, Office Manager
When I was younger I would get turned on by Jackie Collins novels. The women always seemed to be on top of things and in control. I found this gave me confidence. My current partner is my first and he has taught me everything I know. We have been together twelve years and we are still learning and enjoying it! I have recurring fantasies about being grabbed from behind and a man having sex with me. I am unable to turn around, so I'm not one hundred per cent sure if it's my fiancé or not! However, most of the time I prefer to be in control of the situation.

Angelica, 18, Student

One thing I've always found quite sexy in films is when the woman is wearing her boyfriend's clothes, e.g. his baggy shirts or jumpers, and then they make love. Lesbian scenes are a turn-on now, although I would not want to experience such things in reality. I find the fun is in the imagining. I also find a woman's body more arousing in general than a man's body. I can relate to it and imagine how she feels when she is with a man in films, etc.

My favourite fantasy takes place when I am older – about thirty. It's been a hard day, I've been in and out of the law courts (I want to be a legal executive) and I'm on my way home. I have to catch the train, which is quite full; there are about four people standing in my carriage. My neck aches, so I begin to rub it to soothe the aching. Then I feel gentle kisses around my neck, but the person somehow seems familiar so I don't turn around. I just smile and enjoy it. The other people on the train are not paying any attention at this point. Then the man's hands become a little more secure around my waist and they slowly move up until they are caressing my breasts through my thin blouse. I become more and more excited and the other passengers start to take more notice. My blouse is then undone to reveal a skimpy white bra and he starts to pull up my skirt to reveal matching panties and suspenders.

He is now obviously aroused as I can feel his erection on my bottom. I have still not turned around to look at him as he finds my hole and inserts his fingers. He expertly teases me until my juices drip down the palm of his hand; he then inserts his penis from behind until I cannot take any more of him. He then slowly withdraws and repeats this movement so that I can feel every ridge of his dick as he slides in and out of me. All the time, I'm aware of everybody else on the train watching closely. This heightens my arousal and makes me come as I grind against his shaft. As we finish, he pulls me upright and kisses my neck again, then he runs his hands down my body. As I compose myself, I turn to kiss him, but he has gone and I never know who he is, yet there is nothing about him that makes me feel as though I should be scared.

Lisa, 23, Occupation Unknown
I fantasise about once a day or more. Most of the fantasies have recurring themes, although they often take place in different surroundings with different people. When I was younger, I was too embarrassed to discuss sexuality and I felt I was being perverted if I thought of sex or felt sexual. It was a case of 'I'm female therefore I find men attractive'. They had to be men a good few years older than myself, and they had to have a history. I would never have had the confidence to take on a virgin and lead the way!

I have a couple of favourite fantasies. One is of slowly exposing my breasts to some of the old perverts who come into the supermarket – eyeing them up and watching their reaction as I strip off in front of them, tantalising them, playing with myself but never touching them. Most of the old dears think I'm as sweet as icing sugar and I would love to shock them, fulfilling some of their fantasies.

I have another favourite theme and that is of being stimulated by two or three different people at some kind of ceremony, where I am tied to a table and helpless to do anything about it. It is as though it is a set ritual, therefore I know nothing painful or unpleasant will happen to me. There are always a lot of people watching around the edges of the hall where this takes place. My third theme is of standing in a crowded underground train. I am wearing a short skirt, suspenders, stockings and high heels – all black. My bottom is hovering in front of a thirty-something family man. I know he is looking at it, wondering what exactly is under my skirt. I bend down and whisper in his ear, 'Touch me.' He tentatively places his hands on my thighs. There is such a crowd that no one can see what is happening. His hands wander up my thighs to the top of my stockings. He tickles the tops of my thighs and, as I think he is about to slip a finger between my legs, he grabs a buttock in each hand and kneads them. I am standing, holding on to the handrails near the roof.

My breasts are pushed up inside my leather jacket. I unzip the jacket slightly to allow the older man standing in front of me a first-class view as my nipples almost peep out from my Wonderbra. He is transfixed. He leans into me, and I can feel the stiffness in his trousers. Meanwhile, the seated man has taken wild delight in the fact that I am wearing no pants. He is gently rubbing my clit, making me desperate to feel him inside me. I bend over slightly and he can see right up my skirt. He can't resist. His nose presses against my anus as I feel his tongue lapping at my juices. The old man, who looks like a very respectable businessman about to draw his pension, forces his face into my cleavage and tries to release my nipples from the bra with his tongue.

By this time the train has stopped at several stations and the carriage is almost empty. Only the three of us remain, plus a young, beautiful dark-haired female, who is watching us intently. She is fondling her nipples through her thin blouse. The man behind me is about to stand up with his trousers down and plunge his cock deep inside me when the woman walks up and takes my hands. She places them on her breasts. I rip open her blouse to reveal two large, round, brown breasts. The two men stand back and watch as I fondle them and kiss them. They are magnificent. The younger man has reached his peak. He needs to climax. He pushes my skirt up round my waist and pulls me roughly on to his prick. This brings on a long, hard climax for both of us. I pull the woman towards me and unzip her tight denims.

Still sitting on my gentleman friend, I pull her trousers to her knees. She is wearing a crisp, white lace G-string. I pull this down and start to lick at her little bud, kneading her buttocks with my hands. My breasts are pressed up against her thighs and the feeling is sensational. I can feel another climax growing in my belly. The old man has pulled his prick out of his trousers. He is behind the dark woman, rubbing it against her bottom, pulling at her tits with his hands. She moans loudly as I explore her with my fingers and bring her to an earth-shattering climax, while the old man spurts his warm release all over her fleshy buttocks. We all refasten our various articles of clothing without saying a word. In our heads we all know we will meet again next week on the 22.47.

Chris, 37, Art Teacher
I am on a long train journey in one of the old-fashioned carriages that have bench seats with overhead luggage racks. I am feeling really horny and am bored with reading the newspaper. I am dressed very smartly in executive clothes as I'm on my way to a conference. At one stop a group of seven or eight schoolboys aged about fifteen or sixteen get into the carriage I had to myself. They are all nice-looking and wearing uniform. They are not with their teacher. He has gone to the buffet carriage. As soon as they are seated they begin to make crude sexual comments about me. One of the boys – the ringleader – is rubbing his already bulging crotch, saying he would like to fuck me and then the others could have their turn. He gets a porno mag out of his school bag and starts showing me pictures,

asking would I like to pose like the women in the magazine. He gets his cock out and begins unashamedly masturbating with the porno mag open on the seat beside him. I protest, saying they are too young to be reading such stuff, but the ringleader ignores my falsely moralising comments and, instead, pulls me up from my seat and pushes me against the door. He rips my jacket off and shoves his hands up my skirt to find I'm wearing stockings. He gets one or two of the others to feel me up, asking if I'm wet and if they would like to shoot their loads into me. I pretend to be outraged but the ringleader's crude remarks are making me desperate for their cocks.

I am grabbed and my arms are held apart as all the boys take turns in touching my tits and between my legs. The ringleader has to keep pulling them off me, as he wants to be in there first. I keep saying that they are not going to get away with it and that it will be rape, but they say they're going to rape me anyway and I'll love it because I'm really just a filthy slut. My knickers are pulled off and I'm thrown on to the floor between the seats. One boy makes me suck on his cock while the others begin masturbating and saying obscene things. The ringleader starts wanking himself off in front of me and is determined to make it last. The boy whose cock I have in my mouth begins to pump more violently and says he's going to spunk into me. After he's finished and my face is full of come, the ringleader holds me down by my neck and pushes his big cock roughly into me. They've all still got their uniform ties and shirts on. I try to get up – to show I really don't think I should submit to their sexual abuse – but they are too strong and I don't have a chance. The ringleader is telling me he's never been so turned on and he's really enjoying fucking someone who looks like one of his teachers. He makes me suck his cock, too, and then turns me over and takes me from behind while the other boys wank themselves into a frenzy at the sight of my wet cunt. By the time they've all finished, I'm covered in the young men's spunk. Then their teacher enters the carriage . . .

Linda, 27, Nurse
I like fantasising about various situations, such as hitching a ride or being taken over a desk or having sex in a closet at work. I used to be aroused when wearing satin underwear and having sex in the house while my parents were in. Making love to the person I am in love with is a powerful turn-on. These days I like to fantasise about having sex with two men. I like to imagine sex with good-looking bosses and being aroused by a man who can stimulate me to come just with his lips and tongue.

In my favourite fantasy I am hitching a ride. I am wearing a short skirt and a skimpy blouse. In this fantasy I'm a size twelve (I am larger than average in real life). A lorry driver pulls up and I run and jump into his cab. As soon as I get in we both know there is an instant attraction. He is dark and muscular with stubble (as he has been driving a while). We chat for a while but all the time I feel him undressing me with his eyes. I notice a bulge in his jeans, getting bigger and bigger. The fly on his jeans is now bursting. I offer to unbutton his jeans to release it. As I unbutton his fly, it springs out. I cannot believe my eyes at the size of it. It's so big that I don't know what I am going to do with it, so I become very quiet. I keep watching it out of the corner of my eye as he is driving.

He asks me to change gear for him but, instead of taking hold of the gear stick, I take hold of his throbbing cock. (I'm so wet at this point.) It twitches at my touch. I slip off my blouse and hitch up my skirt. I'm not wearing any knickers. I climb over and mount his

24

cock while he is still driving. I ride away; all the time
he continues to drive, because I won't let him stop. His
jeans are rubbing my clit and I begin to come. When
he feels my contractions on his cock, he also comes.
Once we've sorted ourselves out, we reach my desti-
nation and I will never see that throbbing cock again,
which only adds to the pleasure of it.

Kara, 24, Unemployed
I love men in uniforms – army, navy or airforce. I like
to imagine undressing them to find a muscled body
underneath.

I have a favourite fantasy and it goes like this: I meet
up with a stranger – a soldier at the local airport. We
take one look at each other and we just click. We
decide to take a drive to the country. As we are driving
down a country lane, we end up at a country pub/
hotel. Once he has registered us we go up to the room.
It has a four-poster bed, a big log fire and a bottle of
champagne beside the bed. As he closes the door, I go
out to the balcony to look at the woods. He follows me
and puts his hands on my shoulders and guides me
back into the room. He gently moves his hands down
my arms and suddenly pulls me back towards him. I
am now resting in his arms; he starts to kiss my neck
and as he undoes my blouse he turns me around. I feel
his hands on my breasts and we now move over to the
bed. He lays me down.

As I start to undo his shirt, he stops and undresses
himself. Then he climbs on top of me and we have a
deep and tender kiss and make mad, passionate love.
In the small hours he drives off as if nothing has
happened. When I finally awake, there is a note and a
rose saying he had the best time of his life.

Janine, 34, Air Stewardess
I always used to fantasise about rock stars such as
Marc Bolan and Queen. It must have been my 'rough

men' fantasy, which was just beginning. I learnt about sex from *Cosmopolitan* magazine and Jackie Collins novels, then I found a copy of *The Sensuous Woman* in the library and learnt everything overnight! These days I love truckers, bikers, cowboys and lumberjacks, etc. I like dirty talk and a certain amount of attitude. I don't like being wined and dined or treated like a lady. I prefer porno movies and magazines. I also really get off on explicitly sexual books.

There are recurring themes in my fantasies and they run from rape, group sex and exhibitionism to anal sex, lesbianism and anonymous sex with strangers. In my fantasy I'm driving up the motorway in an open-top sports car. It's a hot and humid summer evening and I've taken off my underwear to cool down. All I'm wearing is a short, tight skirt and a white silk blouse. As I drive towards the setting sun, I entertain myself by checking out the truckers as I pass them. I always do this to stop the boredom setting in on long journeys. There's a bastard of a driver in one of these lorries now, and every time I try to pass him he accelerates to stop me getting by. But I love a game of cat and mouse, so I decide to just cruise along beside him for a mile or two.

As I pull level with his side window I glance up into his wing mirror to get a look at him. What I see takes my breath away and instantly sets my imagination working overtime. He's gorgeous. I see that he's shirt-less, bronzed and well muscled, just the way I like men. His hair is dark and glossy with a slight wave, and it hangs just below his shoulders. He has a neatly trimmed full moustache and beard and I can see that he has a perfect pair of sparkling green eyes. This man is my dream lover come to life. I am totally unaware of the road speeding away and of how long I've been watching this guy, when he grins at me and runs his hand through his hair in a gesture of pure flirtatiousness. It startles me and suddenly I want him really badly. I can feel my pussy starting to throb and dampen, yet I have no idea how or even if I can make this happen. A few miles further on and I'm driving in the glow of his tail lights. My left hand is between my legs, leisurely stroking my clit in slow, gentle circles. Despite the warmth of the night air, my nipples are pressing hard against my shirt as I get more and more aroused. I know there is a service area approaching and I start to wonder if I can lure him off with me. Then my prayers are answered; his left indicator starts to flash. I have no choice but to follow.

The service area is brightly lit and coachloads of day-trippers are wandering about drinking Coke and eating crisps. I realise there is overnight parking for HGVs and that's where he's heading. Oh hell, what if I've got it all wrong? I think. What if he doesn't even realise that I'm behind him? He comes to a halt and his lights go off just as I park two or three spaces to his right. I see him jump down from the cab and stretch. His muscular body looks even better than I had imagined. He looks over to me and I can't decide if he smiles or not, then he turns and walks to the other side of his rig. The seconds pass as slowly as hours. What do I do now? My heart is almost bursting out of my chest, I'm so scared, but the heat and wetness between my legs has a stronger control over my actions and so, shaking, I step out of my car. I walk behind the truck, trying to look as though I'm on my way somewhere else. Then, as I pass by, I hear a deep, husky and surprisingly soft voice say, 'I was beginning to think you had changed your mind.'

I turn to see him sitting on the bottom step of the passenger doorway and, as our eyes meet, he stands up and walks towards me. The top two buttons of his jeans are undone, as are the laces of his boots. I can see a fine line of hair growing in the centre of his chest and leading down below the waistband of his jeans. God, how I want to run my tongue through that hair! When he reaches me, I'm afraid my knees are going to give way; I'm afraid that he'll see the moisture that's beginning to run down my thighs. But he smiles a reassuring smile and tells me, 'Well, we can't fuck here in the open,' and turns back to the lorry. It's so coarse and blatant that I almost come there and then, but a passing truck's lights shine on me and I move to follow the man into the shadows.

For some reason, I try to speak and say, 'I don't normally do things like this. I don't want you to think I'm a . . . a . . .' He finishes the sentence for me: 'What? A slut? Well, whatever you are, you're really sexy. Come here.' It's a demand, and I can't help but obey. I step right next to him and he pulls me hard against his body as his mouth crushes against mine, forcing my lips open with his own, pushing his tongue into my mouth as his hands grab big handfuls of my fleshy ass cheeks. He breaks away from me and turns me around as he tells me to get in, and I step up two huge steps until my waist is level with the shabby vinyl seat. His hands move up the backs of my knees until his fingers creep under the hem of my skirt. Still they push upwards, raising the material as they go, exposing my thighs and finally my naked bottom. 'Don't move,' he orders. At that moment I feel his tongue on my goose-pimpled flesh, a moan of sheer pleasure comes from my throat and I can't help but push back at him. He sucks a mouthful of my bottom into his mouth, his teeth closing on it with just the right amount of pressure, his tongue lashing at me. I feel so wanton and lewd; he makes me feel like a whore and I love it, abandoning myself to the wonderful sensations created by the grip of his fingers and the bite of his teeth.

I spread my thighs a little wider for him, displaying my most secret flesh, showing him how wet he's made me, how ready I am to feel him inside me. As his thumbs prise my ass cheeks even wider apart, my knees tremble in anticipation of feeling a finger or tongue enter me. But he holds me there on the edge, his fingers burning into my flesh as he inspects my asshole in a way that makes me feel embarrassed and ashamed. 'Please . . .' I don't want to beg but my resistance is so low now. My bottom is quivering with desire and my pussy is aching and heavy, desperate for some kind of friction on my clit or the feeling of being filled up which would so easily bring me to orgasm. 'Please,' I moan again. He just sniggers to himself and asks me, 'Please what? You're gonna have to tell me what it is you want, lady.' I summon all my nerve and say, 'Please, just help me to come.' I don't have to ask him twice. Instantly he shoves his pointed, firm tongue as far as it will go into my tight little ass pucker, drilling it back and forth roughly, his facial hairs chafing my delicate membranes. It's too much for me; I reach back and pull his hair, rubbing myself back against his face, grinding hard against his mouth. But he senses how close my orgasm is and, laughing, steps away from me, before pulling me back on to the tarmac to stand in front of him. Once again, he turns me around to face him and I sit on the lowest step, my skirt around my waist, hand between my legs, as I watch him unbutton his jeans. He pulls his cock free and strokes it a few times, posing for me in a cocky way. But he has every right to be proud. It's beautiful, not too long, but really thick, circumcised with a huge purple head that's just begging to be licked. He reaches out and grabs my hair, roughly tangling his fingers behind my head as he forces my mouth on to his prick. But I'm more than willing and he gasps aloud as I swallow it down in one long motion, his cock head pushing at the back of my throat. My tongue flicks across the sensitive ridge and probes at his tiny little pee hole before I close my lips around him again. I can smell his sweat and the musky aroma of his arousal and it only adds to my excitement as my head bobs up and down, the pace increasing now. Both his hands move to the back of my head, holding me in a vice-like grip as he really starts to pump and thrust, fucking my mouth with such force I almost gag. I can feel my lips bruising and burning, my saliva running freely over his shaft, mixing with the salty pre-come that's flooding on to my tongue.

Suddenly, he releases me, roughly throwing me around and slamming me against the side of the lorry. I start to be a little afraid, but the fear just turns me on even more. Bracing myself against one of the huge black rubber tyres, I turn my head and watch him over my shoulder. He has hold of his cock but, as he catches my eye, he spits crudely into the palm of his hand and smears the spit all around the swollen purple head. As he moves up behind me I part my legs more, sticking my ass out at him, bending my legs a little, displaying myself so immodestly as I wait to feel his cock enter my cunt. I gasp in surprise as I feel, I think, two fingers go up my bottom. Oh God, no, not that! I've never enjoyed anal sex. Please, not that, not now, not like this. I sob, half in fear, half in animal-like excitement, as he twists his fingers deep inside me. I can feel his mouth at my ear and I'm vaguely aware that he's talking real dirty to me, calling me a slut, a whore, a dirty bitch. As he pulls his fingers out, I feel empty, but not for long. His prick presses insistently at my anal opening. Instinctively my muscles tense against the onslaught, but he tells me, 'Push out, push out.' Despite myself, I do what he asks, and I feel him push a little way inside. The head pops past my tight ring of muscle and he holds still for a moment, allowing me to get used to his size.

His hand comes round the front of me and slips between my legs. For the first time he touches my clit, pinching it and rolling it between his fingertips. Without realising it, I begin to push my bottom down on to his cock, and I want it buried deep inside me. He responds by plunging into me as hard and as deep as he can. He almost lifts me off the ground with each thrust of his pelvis. With his free hand he again wraps my hair around his fingers, pulling my head back hard so that my back arches in an almost impossible curve. Then, without coming out of me even an inch, he turns us both around. He drags me, impaled on his prick, to the doorway again and perches himself on the lowest step, lifting me into his lap to straddle him, my feet barely reaching the ground. I start to lever myself up and down, riding his cock hard, in an attempt to release the unbearable sexual tension that's been gathering inside me for more than an hour now. I sense that he's close to coming, too; his grunting in my ear getting more urgent. He reaches both hands between my thighs, holding my legs wider apart, bouncing me in his lap. Then he starts to rub my clitoris again and shoves three fingers way up inside my cunt. With him penetrating me in both places, I'm pushed over the edge. My orgasm is so intense it's almost too much for me. I writhe on his cock, slamming my body down hard on him, crying tears with the release, as my juices pour over his hands. But he keeps on fingering me; he keeps pressing his swollen cock higher into my bottom until I start to ache.

How can he have held off coming for so long? Again, without slipping out of me, he stands us both up and forces me to bend forward from the waist. Holding my hips fast he changes the pace and starts to fuck my ass fast and shallow. He raises his hand and brings it down hard on my flesh. The sharp sting makes me sob again. 'You like that, don't you, bitch? Huh? You like to feel my hand on your juicy ass.' One last time he slaps me, and I can feel the generous flesh of my bottom quivering and turning pink under his administrations. The sheer humiliation, the way he's making me feel so cheap and slutty, starts a pulsating in the depths of my groin and I know I'm going to come again.

At last I feel his thighs tighten, feel him grip me even more firmly and ram his cock all the way home inside me. Even through my own second orgasm I sense his come splashing against the inner walls of my virgin passage, churning and squelching with every thrust. It seems to last several minutes, and it's not until another set of headlights passes over us that we catch our breath and straighten up. He slips out of me, his come immediately dripping down my thigh, and I watch as he simply stuffs his soft cock back inside his jeans. He says nothing, only adding to my humiliation as I realise my skirt is still twisted round my waist, and both my breasts are exposed through my torn shirt. Embarrassed, I attempt to rearrange my clothing, then I hear his door slam shut. That's it. It's over. He's gone.

Well, that's today's version anyway. I vary this fantasy in length and content depending on my mood, but it's always a trucker, and it's always anal. Sometimes I have sex with his buddies afterwards, both male and female. Thanks for giving me the opportunity to write all this down. I hope it might give pleasure to others.

Dana, 24, Process Worker
I quite often fantasise about science fiction scenarios such as being in a spaceship. I also like imagining myself with my favourite actors and pop stars. When I was younger I found a couple of my dad's videos and got very turned on. I have been very slow to discover my sexuality although I am definitely heterosexual. I had my first orgasm when I was an Ann Summers party organiser a couple of years ago and decided to experiment. I feel much more complete now. Black

Lace books never fail to get me in the mood. Stephen Baldwin, the actor, sends me weak at the knees whenever I see him or even hear his voice. He is in the film *Threesome* which is very good. I tend to just start and let my imagination go wild.

Here is a fantasy I enjoyed. I'm walking through a shady wood alone when a man pops out from behind a tree and stands in front of me. He isn't particularly handsome, but he's rugged and has an air of badness about him. I can't help being attracted but don't show it. He pushes me up against a tree, unlaces the front of my dress and exposes my breasts.

I don't really struggle but I don't help him, either. Then, with one hand, he pulls up my dress at the back and pulls at my pants. He then brings his hand round to the front and puts a finger inside me and moves his hand to one of my breasts. I am now breathing heavily and he unzips his jeans and pulls my pants to the floor. He kneels down with both hands on my nipples and his mouth on my clitoris. He brings me to orgasm and then enters me with his penis. He has me forcefully and fast against the tree. He hasn't removed any of his clothes. He looks at me without a word and gives a sly mocking smile and disappears, leaving me standing exposed and alone.

Karen, 32, Home Carer
I love the idea of sex in exotic places with my husband, sex with more than one man, sex with men and women and sex with just women. I have become very sexual now and can read sex into most things; therefore lots of situations turn me on.

Here is my favourite fantasy. I am on my way into town to shop. Driving along the two-lane road, I notice a man looking at me. He gets into the lane behind me and follows me to the supermarket. Suddenly he is standing in front of me. He looks at me with passion

and says, 'I want you now!' I follow him and we go
into the disabled toilet. He turns to me and kisses me.
Then his hands stroke me everywhere. He peels off my
clothes and I am naked. He is still dressed. He makes
me kneel on the loo, then he kneels on the floor behind
me. He starts to lick and suck me and I come and
come. He takes his clothes off. His body is hairy. He
sits on the toilet and pulls me on top of him. I ride his
cock while he sucks my nipples. I try not to scream.
We come together then get dressed. We walk out; he
goes one way and I go the other. I never see him again.

Ella, 23, Administrator
In my fantasies I am always dominated by male or
female lovers, friends and neighbours, etc. I used to
have similar fantasies involving male or female dominance of a female who is forced into sexual situations.
Alien abductions, princes and princesses and servant
girls also featured strongly.

Here is my favourite fantasy. A young girl works in
a multistorey office complex as a secretary. She doesn't
know it but she has caught the eye of a few fellow
workers. She is in work early today, alone on her floor.
She needs a break; she started work at 5.30 a.m. So,
walking silently down a long corridor, she slips into
the ladies' toilets. No need to lock any doors, she
thinks, as her fellow workers won't be in for another
two hours. As she seats herself on the toilet, her need
to void her urine passes, so she slips her fingers inside
herself, making them wet. She then proceeds to mois-
ten her clit. She pictures somebody, anybody, caressing
her nipples then licking their way down to her fine
thatch of dark hair. He probes his tongue deep inside;
smelling, tasting and teasing. With her eyes closed, she
nears climax as her fingers rub faster. The ladies' room
door opens silently. The intruder is aware of the girl's
presence but she is not aware of him. Carefully placing

a hand over the girl's eyes, a voice says, 'Keep them closed and enjoy; let me pleasure you like no other has.' Her fantasy is fulfilled, though she knows not who has fulfilled it. Maybe she'll come in early again tomorrow.

Angela, Age unknown, Housewife

I think about bondage, sex in the open, rape, sex with a stranger and making love to another woman. The things that turn me on are erotic books, men's magazines, being tied up, my partner's body, the thought of making love with him, experimenting with sexual positions, thinking of new ways to satisfy my partner and giving and receiving oral sex. In the early days, when I was discovering my sexuality, the things that turned me on were watching pornographic videos, seeing other people having sex and tight jeans.

In my favourite fantasy I am lying in bed with the moonlight streaming through the window. A tall dark stranger walks into my room. He comes over to me and ties my hands to the bed with a pair of black stockings. He then begins to kiss me all over, but not my breasts or vagina or clitoris. I begin to writhe in anticipation of what's to happen. He then begins to suckle my breasts, bringing me close to orgasm, but not quite there. His fingers roam my body, brushing my clitoris slightly. He does this for a while, and then he begins to kiss my clitoris and then my right foot and ankle. He works his way up my leg. He kisses my clitoris again and this time begins to lick it. My orgasms don't stop; just as one finishes, another is nearly there.

He then stands up and slowly undresses and, as he takes off his trousers, his penis springs up – it is enormous! He slowly lowers himself on to me and slides inside me. The shock of his penis inside me sends me off on another orgasm. He takes me slowly, sending me higher and higher with each orgasm. When he finally comes it knocks me over the edge with the biggest orgasm I've ever had. My eyes start to close and I can feel his hand untying my wrists. I then fall asleep completely satisfied.

Jayne, 27, Occupation Unknown

When I was younger, older men (but not too old!) or men of a different race were a turn-on. Also, a Wonder-bra of my aunt's that was two sizes too small for me. These days, I think about having sex with a woman or with an occult leader. Sex in public places or with strangers is arousing, as are large, fat dicks.

My recurring fantasy is of being fucked by a truck driver in the back of his truck or by a stranger in a public swimming pool. The truck driver, too, would be a total stranger and not necessarily attractive. I would like to be hitchhiking and be picked up by a truck driver. He would see that I was tired and ask if I wanted to take a nap in the back of his truck. I would fall asleep and would be woken by the truck stopping. He would then climb in the back with me. He would stand/sit by me and show me how turned on he was by seeing me in my underwear. I would take down his zip and suck his throbbing cock. He would rip my knickers off and start licking my wet lips whilst unveiling my ample breasts so he could massage them with his big hands.

He would then kiss me so that I could taste myself on him, while he finds my entrance with his now-bulging hot dick. When he's inside, he sucks my tits while pulling on my hair and pumping in and out of my wet crevice. I'd like him to be biting my nipples as well as sucking them. He would then ask if he could come all over my big breasts. I'd oblige. He would shoot his load all over me and rub it into my soft skin.

We would lie down together for a while until he's ready to start again.

Fay, 22, Student
I think about young boys I know; boys I've had a brief sexual encounter with or a boy in particular that I want to see again. A few years ago riding horses (black stallions) was a turn-on, as was power and mastery. I like young men of seventeen to nineteen years old; and beautiful and sexy classic-looking boys, such as public schoolboys and boys with fast cars.

I think sex on the first night is a morally correct procedure. Waiting is a false pretence if you want to shag each other desperately. Most of my fantasies are based on real life. Only the other night I was lucky enough to pull a gorgeous eighteen-year-old. Unfortunately I had my period and couldn't have sex with him. I was gutted! We had an erotic night, however. I sucked him off. He had a tattoo of a bulldog on his back; he was to die for! I'm so sad because we had a wonderful night and then, in the morning, he didn't seem keen to see me again. I hate it when you have a taste of something beautiful and he's gone for dust in the morning! I want sex every night of the week and on call. I want young boys as sex servants!

Jacqui, 32, Shop Manageress
I once had a dirty phone call but, instead of feeling scared, it turned me on so powerfully that I brought myself off thinking about it for weeks afterwards. It gave me fuel for new fantasies, which is always welcome! In reality, not much happened, except that I didn't slam the phone down when the guy was talking to me. He told me he had 'nine inches' and asked me the usual stuff, like, 'What colour knickers are you wearing?' It was him who rang off first! In my fantasy I take things further and get him to tell me what he really wants to do. I like to think that he is a real sex

maniac, and has to wank off about five times a day. I help him to achieve this by talking dirty to him on the phone. I get him to tell me how he has to visit peep-shows and sleazy video booths to get rid of his hard-ons. I like to imagine him pumping his cock really hard. It excites me to think he may be dangerous, but I know I will be safe because I'm as filthy as he is, and it's only naive, easily shocked women who are at risk. We gradually up the ante: he tells me things I have to keep secret, I tell him about the dirtiest things I've ever done. By only conversing by phone, I can imagine that he is young and good-looking; I wouldn't want to meet him in real life in case he was grubby. I like my men to be really clean, physically.

Chapter Three

Bountiful Lust: Puritans and Libertines, the Group-Sex Fantasy

And priests in black gowns were walking their rounds,
And binding with briars my joys and desires.
                    William Blake, *The Garden of Love* (1788)

Group sex conjures up images of writhing bodies in various states of undress; orgies where people feast lustily on fruit and flesh, and give vent to their lascivious desires. It's the quintessential recreation in any Bacchanalia, and has inspired the imagination of many artists, including Delacroix, Ingres, Rubens and Hogarth. The basic principle behind the orgy is that, if something is good, multiply it and reap your reward! There's nothing new about the idea of group sex but, like same-sex love, it has courted a controversial history. It's a categorically unchristian act of defiance; one cannot use the excuse of procreation to defend the pleasure. Group sex is the logical progression of profligacy; it's what happens when things 'get out of hand'.

It has long been in the interests of the state and the

Church to maintain a close scrutiny over the antics of its subjects. While a blind eye could be turned away from gentlemen of a certain rank or priests indulging themselves, it didn't do for the lower classes to be seen idling and fornicating while there was work to be done. Despite this, for a brief period in the eighteenth century, Europe saw an era of sexual freedom that was to some extent justified by the new sciences that emerged during the Age of Enlightenment. It was a period of welcome rationality after the oppression of the Puritan era, although the emancipation of women would have to wait another couple of centuries before being allowed on the agenda for social change. There was, however, a downside to the freedom. The unbridled licentiousness that erupted meant that venereal disease became rife, and someone had to take the blame for all the unseemly behaviour and physical malady. It was not going to be the lord of the manor, however. Where you found rakes and Casanovas, you also found women of ill repute. Temptation has traditionally been given a female form. The devil comes in the guise of a woman. And if you are weak and succumb to this temptation, you will have to pay the price. Earthly pleasures will pass, and you will be left with the pox and death.

It doesn't take too great a leap of the imagination – or flourish of the brush on canvas – to transform a merry-making Bacchanalia into a devilish Saturnalia, where expressions of pleasure contort into twisted grimaces and the bounty of the human form becomes overripe. Where there is paradise, there is also venom, as the Bible and Western art continue to tell us, and if we waste our time in idolatry and on the pursuit of sins of the flesh, we will come to no good end.

But punishment hasn't always been the message of bountiful sex. The earliest depictions of orgiastic indulgence were positive. It was a popular pastime among the privileged members of Roman society, while the Ancient Greeks revelled in the cult of Dionysus. The art of this period, much of it dating from the sixth century BC, features priapic satyrs and maenads (female worshippers of Dionysus) frolicking and fornicating. One famous piece of Greek pottery of the time depicts a smiling woman watering a garden of phalluses, implying that having access to more than one penis is a good thing. The murals and mosaics of Pompeii are resplendent with scenes of ecstatic coupling, and multiple copulation is the ubiquitous feature in any scene of happiness and celebration in the art of the period. Being virile or potent was a sign of good health. The erect penis or female figure displaying her genitals (later known as the Sheela-na-gig in Celtic art) was used as an amulet to ward off bad spirits. Penile wind chimes and water bowls were favourite household artefacts in Ancient Rome and Greece, and a huge tumescent member was widely recognised as a good-luck charm.

Eastern art, too, saw its own form of eroticism, and early Indian carvings are alive with voluptuous figures finding joy through their own or their partners' bodies. Even cave paintings feature men and animals sporting erections, and the palaeolithic goddess figurines show the exaggerated female form, pregnant, heavy breasted, fecund. Museums across the world have hidden collections of archeological artefacts they believe too indecent for display, such as the first-century Peruvian figures of human males performing anal sex. The earliest images of sex are in many ways the most honest and cheerful, and our ancestors seem to have been at ease with their sexuality and their bodies. So what happened?

Since the dawn of the Christian era, and for well over a millennium prior to the Age of Enlightenment, the natural process of sex has become increasingly tainted with notions of evil. A brief look at history is useful in establishing how pleasure got bound up with guilt. The concept of original sin, that we are all born out of lust, is part of the doctrine of Roman Christianity that came to Great Britain in the sixth century. To have carnal knowledge was to invite the devil and to re-enact the Fall of Man. To gain control over the pagan people of Britain the missionaries preached fear and loathing, and nowhere more vigorously than around aspects of sex.

The idea of *celebrating* each other's bodies was anathema to the po-faced patriarchs. In the year AD 597 Pope Gregory ordered St Augustine to travel to Britain in order to restyle the ways of the British Church in the manner of the Roman original. The Angles and Saxons who had entered Britain in the 5th century were seen as a savage race, and Augustine was very wary of meeting the Saxon warlord-king Ethelbert. Pope Gregory wanted to see a smooth shift from paganism to Christianity, but some of his patriarchal missionaries saw it differently, and it wasn't too long before heavy-handed tactics were being employed to subdue paganism and bring about a successful conversion. A few zealots conveniently called the indigenous Angles' and Saxons' religion devil worship. They preached that their heathen life would result in being consumed by the infernal fires of hell at death.

They took old fertility gods and turned them into cloven-hoofed devils; they took the festivals of the ancient pagan calendar, such as Eostre and Yule, and made them Easter and Christmas. They built churches on the site of sacred burial grounds and temples, and appropriated their gods and goddesses and turned them into Christian saints. They literally put the fear of God into the pagans.

This may seem irrelevant to a book on women's sexual fantasies. But what happened all that time ago was to have lasting repercussions on British attitudes to sex. The pagan culture was in a large part a goddess-worshipping culture; the Earth Mother was represented in all aspects of the landscape. Fecundity and fertility was cyclical, and the sacred systems dictated by nature were seen as female in manifestation; for instance, the lunar calendar having the same number of days as a woman's menstrual cycle. The sky god of Roman Christianity was the polar opposite of an earth goddess, ergo, eradicating the heathen beliefs needed to demonise the female. The tolerance and kindness of Jesus's teachings were somehow transformed into a rigid doctrine that forbade pleasure; that preached damnation of unbelievers, and terrified ordinary folk.

It took a couple of hundred years to fully convert the pagan Saxons to Christianity but they had a good publicity machine, and the alarming rate at which churches were constructed ensured a wholesale conversion through realising absolute power, starting with the king and working down. Tolerance and kindness are not qualities one associates with the holy men of the Middle Ages. In the thirteenth century St Thomas Aquinas went as far as to declare the sexual act – even between man and wife – a venial sin; the only untainted woman who had ever lived was the mother of Jesus. The fear of the female body became so great that even the concept of the Mother of God's womb being pierced became too risky, and alternative theories as to how the Immaculate Conception took place included the rumour that Mary conceived the Holy Spirit by means of a shaft of light passing into her ear, through which the spirit of God entered her body.

Menstruation became feared and demonised and seen as woman's curse. Aquinas arrogantly suggested that God had made a mistake in creating woman: 'nothing [deficient] or defective should have been produced in the first establishment of things; so woman ought not to have been produced then.'[1] Lutherans at Wittenberg in the 1500s debated whether women were really human beings at all.[2] Orthodox Christians held women responsible for all sin. As the Bible's *Apocrypha* states, 'Of woman came the beginning of sin. And thanks to her, we all must die.'[3] The Christian world became what Monica Sjöö has called 'biophobic': denying and rejecting the natural physical processes and making them taboo. Contrary to Eastern practice of the same period, where Taoist and Tantric teachings taught men to be experts in giving women sexual pleasure, the European male was being told that a sexual woman was a demon, a snake and something to be silenced and feared and locked away. Even childbirth was seen as something to fear. Clerics took this quote from *Genesis* to a sadistic extreme: 'In sorrow shall you bring forth children.' Martin Luther, the founder of Protestantism, declared, 'If a woman grows weary and at last dies from child-bearing, it matters not. Let her die from bearing, she is there to do it.'

The philosopher Pascal noted that men never do evil so completely and cheerfully as when they do it from religious conviction. The four centuries preceding the Age of Enlightenment surely bear out his wise words. The period between the fourteenth and eighteenth centuries have been called the 'burning times', what R. H. Robbins called 'the shocking nightmare, the foulest crime and deepest shame of western civilisation,' [4] where the hysteria around witchcraft resulted in the sanctioned murder of several million people, nearly all women. Their 'crimes' included such innocuous practices as gathering herbs at night, easing women's pain during childbirth, or talking to a cat. The *Malleus Maleficarum*, the handbook for witch-hunters and given blessed authority by the pope of the time, carried instructions for the torturing of women with no fixed limit to barbarity.

With that kind of paranoia hanging over ordinary people, it is no surprise that the pendulum was set to swing so far in favour of sexual liberalism. When the Age of Enlightenment dawned over a miserable Puritan Europe, it offered a way out of one of the worst periods of sexual repression in world history. Scholars became critical of the received authority and the old doctrines and looked for ways to unite the natural with the rational. The idea that man – and not a vengeful God – may be responsible for his own destiny came as a great relief. This period saw the emergence of erotic emancipation and the profligacy that swept across all ranks of European society became the talking point of the day. Even Christianity got on the bandwagon. The natural desires began to be seen as our God-given right, and to suppress one's appetite was thought of as unhealthy. Look at this statement by the Reverend Daniel Maclauchlan, published in 1735: 'It should be the business of our lives to plant and propagate our kind, and to throw our seed into every fruitful corner. To get it vigorously into the gaping bottom of every sweet-watered vale.'[5]

More notoriously, the Reverend Martin Madan, the chaplain to the London venereal disease hospital, argued in 1780 for the restoration of polygamy, postulating that it would give all women a chance to marry, end prostitution and be an effective cure for male sexual frustration. These men took their lead from scholars such as James Boswell and Samuel Johnson. Sex and health became intimately associated. Erasmus Darwin and many other physicians prescribed lovemaking as a remedy for psychosomatic disorders. However, it was men's health that was seen as being of paramount importance. Women were expected to tolerate male dalliances and turn a blind eye to their husbands' taking of concubines. It is fun to romanticise the bawdy romps of the time, but the sexual liberalism of the libertines was heavily influenced by patriarchal notions of acquisitiveness; of notching scores on the bedposts and discarding the goods once they were soiled.

We are all living under the weight of our ancestors' social mores. Throughout history the pendulum has swung back and forth: from pre-Christian paganism and goddess worship to Augustinian Christianity; from repressive Puritanism and institutionalised misogyny to rational libertinism and erotic emancipation; from Victorian morality and the introduction of obscenity laws (that remain on the statute books) to the permissive society of the 60s, right through to today's postmodern dilemma, where the moral Christian right has linked hands with the pro-censorship feminist.

It's unsurprising that many of our fantasies attempt to redress the balance; to allow ourselves some brief respite from codes of behaviour and rules of all kinds. This is the second largest section in the book, being beaten only by exhibitionism, which itself features fantasies involving multiple partners. There's something life affirming about the group-sex fantasy; a primal thanksgiving for all the pleasure it's possible to have. All mixtures of group sex are there: women with other women in front of their male partners, one woman with lots of men, different racial mixes. A lot of the fantasies involve being watched by someone, usually male, who is desperate to join in or helpless to prevent himself being overcome with desire.

The reality of multi-partnered shenanigans can be all too complex; we might not want to see our husband or wife getting a good seeing to from a stranger who may be younger and prettier or better endowed than ourselves. The ego will persist in reminding us that life is a competitive business, and actively introducing our lover to another sex partner may put our relationship at risk. In the group-sex fantasy our boyfriends and girlfriends don't get jealous, and no one's feelings are hurt. Alternatively, we can imagine ourselves with total strangers, famous people or powerful archetypes. One topical fantasy was submitted by Lela, who imagines herself giving an unnamed president of the United States a blow job at the White House, while his securityguards join in. A lot of group-sex fantasies are about showing off; being desirable to more than one person at the same time and having the best of all worlds. Some of the fantasies remind me of Rabelasian scenarios, particularly Natasha's tale of being on the farm, pushed under the hay cart and having all her favourite things done to her. If your idea of heaven is having a variety of bodies to play with, you will love the fantasies in this section.

Pet, 19, Occupation Unknown

I am nineteen years of age and bisexual, but prefer my own sex to men. I was always a bit of a tomboy and got turned on seeing my friends dressed in the kind of feminine clothes I didn't wear. I also got turned on imagining myself in those clothes. I was sometimes also turned on by watching my friends in the showers, or getting dried by rubbing themselves. These days I haven't lost interest in looking at other girls and like to imagine what they would look like in suspenders and G-strings. I don't really find explicit porn movies sexy, but I like watching dirty films and reading erotic literature.

My favourite fantasy is to meet and have sex with a black couple. She would need to have large, firm tits with large nipples that you would never want to stop sucking and biting. Her cunt would need to be shaved, and have large lips and a prominent clit. To be between those strong muscular thighs with the man's cock pounding into me from behind would be heaven. An ebony and ivory sandwich with me in between would then ensue, followed by a love triangle with me sucking his hard, thick penis. My cunt is being tongued and fingered by the black bombshell; her pink tongue probing and licking, while she herself is being milked by the big black stud. The fantasy is completed by the black couple making out, the girl astride his thighs, with myself, in the meantime, perched over his face, watching his cock pounding piston-like into her hairless cunt. Then I collapse on to him and reach out for her gorgeous melon-like breasts and help her to orgasm as we all come together again.

Nancy, 24, Student
I like to fantasise about a man – and sometimes a woman – whom I happen to have a crush on at that time. He is just the perfect lover and I am exactly as great a lover as he thought I'd be. I kind of play a whole night of passion and wild abandon through in my head and caress myself the way he would. I have this fantasy when I feel lonely or sad. At other times I imagine more kinky stuff and try to come up with new images and ideas as often as I can.

When younger, I adored female bodies in tight, elegant dresses. Angelica Houston as a femme fatale vampire was a particular turn-on. I think the reason is that I feel extremely sexy when I wear black dresses with high heels. Even when I was young I would dress to go out and masturbate before going to the party or whatever. I felt so much more sexy than my normal, boring self. As for people – George Clooney from *ER*, of course! I now find that I am turned on more and more by voices; for example, if a man has a deep, masculine voice with a certain timbre, my knees just go weak!

My current favourite fantasy is set in an imaginary girlfriend's house. We talk and drink some wine. After some time we start caressing each other and openly make out. What I don't know is that she has agreed this with her boyfriend, who is watching the whole scene from the room next door. He strokes himself while he watches us stimulate and suck each other. When we have both orgasmed, we lie there, still entwined. He comes into the room and starts touching us both, first gently fondling, then demanding more and more from our whole bodies. First he wants to sleep with his girlfriend but decides to try something new by sleeping with me. He arouses me, kisses my face, my breasts and my sex, while my friend watches in fascination.

He realises that I am really wet and ready for him. He then enters me, and we both realise that it is perfect. The perfect match. We heave and roll together, totally lost in this overwhelming lust. We forget where we are, we forget my best friend; she is sitting there stunned, watching us. There are only our bodies, our needs. We kiss and our tongues dance to a wild rhythm while our bodies ache to be released. When we are finally spent, we know we will stay together; we have found the missing half.

Tanya, 21, Engineering Student
I like fantasies about group sex, particularly two men and sometimes another woman. Men in uniform, such as policemen or firemen, do it for me, too. These days I love using my vibrator; it's even better when my boyfriend uses it on me. I like buying sexy underwear from Ann Summers parties and I read a lot of erotic fiction.

Here is my current favourite story: It was Friday evening and I had been shopping all day and had treated myself to some new underwear to surprise my boyfriend. It was a really sexy black satin basque, with lots of lace trim, and knickers to match that tied at the sides. When I got out of my bath, I decided to try on all my new underwear. I looked great. I could just imagine my boyfriend's face. Sometimes I really like to spice things up with new underwear or a sex toy. I began to imagine all the things he would do to me. Just as my dream began to hot up, the doorbell went. I grabbed my silk dressing gown and ran downstairs.

I opened the door and who should be standing there but Gary Jackson – the best-looking bloke on earth. He was with a guy called Len, whom I didn't know. I invited them both in, but I couldn't keep my eyes off Gary. He is 26, about six feet three inches with floppy, blond hair and sexy blue eyes and a sexy, fit body. Len isn't bad either; same height as Gary with deep blue eyes.

'Do you want a drink? I've got some cans in the fridge,' I asked. I was starting to feel really turned on, and went into the kitchen. I could feel my nipples going hard, rubbing against my basque. The feeling of arousal was mounting between my legs, the wetness soaking my panties. I put my hand inside my dressing gown, lightly stroking my finger down my body. I then slipped my hand inside my panties and shuddered at my own touch, as my fingers softly rubbed my clit. My sex was wet; I was wishing Gary could be doing this. The start of an orgasm flowed through my body. I slid a finger into my waiting vagina and my juices flowed out. I rubbed my clit a bit harder and leant against the table. Just knowing that Gary and Len could walk in at any moment was even more exciting. My orgasm took over, but my body wanted more. Just as my fingers, wet with my dew, slid in and out of me, Len walked into the kitchen.

A smile spread over his face. 'I can see what you are doing. Do you like touching yourself when you come into the kitchen or is it something else?'

I didn't even feel embarrassed, even though I was still leaning against the table with my legs slightly apart and my hands down my panties. Len walked over to me and touched the top of one of my stockings and slid his finger into the top of it.

'Do you want Gary? Wouldn't you like him to be stroking your clit and licking it, then to take you with his cock and thrust himself into you?' Len said.

I moved my hand from out of my panties. Len knows I want Gary. I tried to get past him but he pushed me back up against the table. He kissed me, gently at first, then more eagerly. His hands were all over my body. He started to kiss my neck and the familiar feeling of arousal started in my womb. Len cupped my breasts in his hands, and my nipples rubbed hard, erect with desire, against my basque. He moved his fingers on to my nipples, gently squeezing them, then more roughly. I gasped as he started to rub himself against my wanting body. I started to push him away.

'What's the matter, babe? Don't you like me doing this?' he asked. Len pulled at my panties, and the sides of them opened easily to reveal my mound. The dew made my sex glisten. Len stroked my clit harder and harder until I could feel my knees weaken. His breathing got faster and he pushed two fingers inside me. I started moving on them as if it was his cock thrusting into me. My love juices were making his fingers shine. His fingers thrust into me harder and faster as I came. My womb pulsated with an orgasm as I looked at Len.

'So, Tanya, now do you want my cock?' asked Len. As he pulled out his fingers, I groaned with disapproval. He winked at me and went back into the other room. I straightened myself up and followed, my knees still weak at the experience.

The TV was getting on my nerves and I went to switch it off. I bent over, then remembered that I hadn't put my knickers back on and my dressing gown only just covered my bottom.

'Tanya, you naughty girl, you're not wearing any knickers,' said Gary. I giggled. I now knew that this was what I really wanted. I was totally horny, and with the drink, I didn't really care.

'Take that silky thing off, honey, so we can see a bit more of you,' said Len.

I undid the belt and took it off teasingly.

'Show me your pussy, babe,' said Gary. I pulled my lips apart, so he could see my stiff clit. I rubbed myself, watching the look of wanting on Gary's face. Gary pushed me down so he was on top of me. He kissed me and forced his tongue inside my mouth. He started to undo my basque and kissed my neck, his hot breath tickling me. As he pulled at my basque, it came away from my firm breasts, now on show. He unclipped the basque from the stockings and pulled the stockings down.

His hands were running wildly all over my body. His long fingers stroked around my breasts. He kissed me again and started to move downwards. His tongue went into my love tunnel, probing deep inside, pushing into me. I began thrusting up against his mouth. I wanted it deeper. He was tasting my juices. Len was watching and I realised that he was naked. He walked over and started to caress my breasts, then he moved his hand towards my pussy and started to rub my clit. I watched Gary get undressed and saw his throbbing hard length. He was so big. He rubbed his cock between his hands and walked over to me. He knelt down beside me. I grabbed his cock and brought my mouth to it. I licked its purple head and took him into my mouth. The size of him made me gag. I wanted to swallow him. As I sucked on him greedily, I felt Len push his cock into my vagina. I felt complete at last. I sucked faster on Gary's cock as Len fucked me harder. Gary moaned as he shot his seed into my mouth. The warm, salty taste of his pleasure slid down my throat.

Len was now pounding so fast and so deep that I moved away from Gary's cock and groaned as my orgasm took me over. Len made one final thrust and he came. I came again when I could feel his cock throb as he shot his sperm into me. I lay on my back totally exhausted, pleased that I could make two men orgasm at once.

Gary smiled and started tossing himself off, so that he could get hard again. I helped him and also helped Len. I was surprised at how quickly they both got hard again.

Len sat on the chair and I bent over him taking his length into my mouth. I opened my legs and Gary moved in between them and entered my wet cunt. He pumped into me and I pumped up and down on Len's cock. I took him out of my mouth and licked up and down Len's cock. I nibbled it, kissed it and ran my tongue all over it.

Gary's fucking started to get faster as his balls bounced off me. I jerked myself backwards to get his shaft even deeper inside me. Len was in my mouth again. He came first, and then Gary. I felt satisfied; my mouth was filled with happiness as my body was filled with ecstasy. I now felt a complete being: fucked by two different men and sucking them both off is something I have never done before, particularly as neither of them are boyfriends. I thought about it as 'sex for fun'.

I was glad I shagged Gary; I'd wanted him for ages. As for Len, he was the perfect stranger – well, sort of. What a dirty girl I am, but who cares; you're only young once!

Magda, 30, Housewife

The idea of sex with several men makes me horny. I also find lingerie and steamy novels erotic. I love seeing my partner take a shower. I like watching him as he washes himself and as he watches me, I am watching him! I have a fantasy that fulfils my sexual needs. Here it is: I am returning home from work and I call into our local pool hall. When I enter there are only five men there. I get a drink when suddenly the biggest man grabs me. He tells me that they need an extra pocket. He lays me on the table, spreads my legs and gently cues the ball between them. When he sees how aroused I am getting he gets harder. His friends come over and join in and we all have a ball of a time!

Caroline, 26, PA and Model
I have several recurring fantasies: threesomes (two women and one man) and the idea of being watched making love. I used to get really turned on by making love in public places and watching films with my partners. The more provocative and exciting the better. I also like reading stories aloud to a partner.

A current fantasy is for my partner to tie me to a dining table and blindfold me. He spends some time touching me very gently, which provokes me. Suddenly he leaves the room. Footsteps return and I feel a tongue licking and sucking my clitoris. A body then climbs above me and the licking alters for a while. I feel hair above my mouth and realise that it is a woman in the 69 position with me, and I cannot move. She brings me off and I enjoy licking her. She then removes my blindfold and I see that a number of other men are there and have watched the whole thing. A couple of these men then take me on the table while I suck my boyfriend's cock. He comes at the same time as the other men and the fantasy ends.

Natasha, 26, Housewife/Carer
I fantasise a few times a month and a favourite is an old boyfriend coming back on to the scene and seducing me, or me seducing him. Anything really can turn me on! I do use erotic fiction and films to get me going

and also mirrors, too. I like to lie on the rug in front of a real fire watching an erotic movie with my boyfriend.

My current favourite starts off as a dream. I'm working on a farm with about four of my ex-boyfriends. There is a lot of hay about and an old cart. One of my exes grabs me from behind and pushes me face down on to some hay under the cart. He starts kissing the back of my neck and back and runs his hands all over my body. All my other exes are working on the farm, oblivious to what is going on. My ex knows just what I like. He takes me from behind and suddenly all my exes are holding me down and doing all my favourite things to me. They take it in turns to pleasure me and make me happy. Then I wake up.

Coral, 23, Clerical Worker
Some of my fantasies are set in hotel rooms; others on country walks and some in a sex shop. A lot of things influenced me when I was young. Books, however, were my main enjoyment, as well as unusual things such as bondage and control freaks. I like to read about or watch all people now: females with females, females with males, but not males together. I am quite open minded, be it S&M, watersports or even animals.

My favourite fantasy takes place in a hotel room. I am alone and bored. I decide to play with myself. While this is going on, the maid enters. She isn't shocked but interested. She takes off her uniform and joins me on the bed, where we get up to everything from licking each other to fisting. We move to the shower and have more fun, including watersports, then back to the bedroom where we start again. We haven't realised but the hotel manager has been watching us all along. He comes out with a huge erection and joins in. I climax as the maid licks me out while the hotel manager is kneeling and coming all over me.

Sometimes, it isn't a hotel manager but a window

cleaner who is helpless outside and can only watch. He comes all over his nice clean window!

Danni, 25, Unemployed
My recurring fantasy is to be seduced by another woman while my husband watches and later joins in. My first boyfriend was highly sexed. In fact, it was sex on impulse. We had sex in every shelter overlooking the beach where we worked at the time. My second boyfriend made me sex mad. While I was living with him he would make me wear sexy underwear to bed. I would wear stockings and suspenders, which made me feel really sexy. We were having sex at least twice a day, and once or twice we were at it all night.

These days I enjoy watching porno films. I like seeing people naked on TV, enjoying themselves and trying all sorts of different positions. I would like a woman who I got on with and I thought was sexy, to live with my husband and I as it would make our marriage better. She could help me cook and clean and, if I was horny, I could jump into bed with her, and if my husband was horny he could as well. If she was horny she could jump into bed with us. But what woman would live with a married couple for a while?

My favourite fantasy goes like this. I am asleep in bed and my husband gets up to go and do something. While he is out, a woman slips into my bed and starts feeling my body all over. She starts to feel between my legs and later goes down to lick me. After a while my husband walks in and enjoys what he sees, quickly throwing off his clothes and joining us. He is lying on his side. I am on my back with my legs over his side and he is screwing me. The girl is bent over his side, licking my clitoris wildly. Then one of my husband's friends turns up and they talk about what has just happened. They both open the bedroom door to watch the girl and I enjoying each other's bodies. I am lying on my back and the girl is on top of me, facing my feet. My husband is fucking the girl doggy-style while I lick her clitoris. In the meantime my husband's mate is giving me what for. We keep swapping around all day.

My husband isn't big on sex, so I guess this won't happen. Then again, I don't know if I would have the nerve, either, so I'll keep reading Black Lace instead!

Kirsty, 38, Office Worker
I like to fantasise that I have been caught masturbating by the window cleaner, butler and maid, etc. I like muscular arms, articles in blue magazines, sexy novels and silky underwear.

Here is my favourite fantasy. I am by the pool of a very wealthy friend, who is very naive regarding sex. I get my breasts from out of my swimsuit and she licks my nipples, slowly at first, and then more forcefully. I show her how wet my vagina is and I insert my vibrator so that she can watch. She sees it slide deeply inside me, then I pull it out and rub it on my swollen clitoris. At that moment her butler is bringing out some drinks. He sees what we are doing and the bulge in his trousers gets bigger and bigger. I offer myself to him by opening my legs wider. He inserts his penis in me. My friend watches with interest. She then touches my clitoris and sucks my nipples hard. I orgasm while she frigs me, sucks me and he fucks me. He then fucks her from behind while I watch in the afterglow of coming.

Jodie, 34, Occupation Unknown
I fantasise dozens of times a day and each fantasy is very different. If there are recurring themes they are based on group sex and wild sex; sometimes things that I wouldn't necessarily do. I also draw from experiences and relationships and imagine people I don't know but would like to; for example, Bjork!

I only recently discovered my bisexuality, although

I've always found women attractive. I've also only just discovered my ability to ejaculate when I come. These days I get very turned on by my girlfriend – we sleep together once a week – and by my male lover, whom I fuck in bed or anywhere we can: in the office, on the stairs, outside, etc. As I said, my fantasies are based around real-life experiences; with my lover and my girlfriend, and sometimes with her husband, too. We play games such as 'wet things' or watersports and have threesomes and foursomes. We enjoy bondage, spanking and lots and lots of hot sex. I like women and men. I have to survive! I am in a sexually unfulfilled marriage and all this is very secret and special. It keeps me sane!

Lois, 22, Housewife

I have fantasies several times a day. They used to be stimulated by sexy books and blue films my father used to have. It was a turn-on to see all the different things that you could do with men and women. I still find films and books a turn-on, but my husband isn't very adventurous sexually so films are usually out of the question. I recently got very turned on by a facial, neck, shoulder and chest massage. I was imagining what would happen if the hands went a little lower on to my breasts.

I often fantasise about having a threesome with two strangers. It's always in different settings, sometimes a massage parlour, sometimes a doctor's surgery or a shop changing room. Two strangers have set up the situation and the woman seduces me first. Then the man appears and either joins us or watches and masturbates himself. Sometimes he takes photographs.

I also fantasise about making love to a woman alone. The settings are always different; sometimes we are bathing together, soaping each other down. Other times we are in bed laughing and joking and one thing leads to another. I don't have just one favourite fantasy, but they usually have a gay theme.

Lorraine, 38, Nursery Nurse

I fantasise a couple of times a week and my main fantasies consist of a relationship with another woman. Also I like my partner to take control. When I was younger, any sexually charged or erotic film turned me on. Just knowing a man wants me, even if nothing happens, is a turn-on. I like the idea of being told what to do. Watching other couples making love in a film or gay and lesbian sex scenes are particularly erotic.

Here is my favourite fantasy. I am buying a very expensive dress and the assistant brings in different ones for me to try. None of them look right, so the supervisor – a very beautiful woman – comes over to help. She says my underwear is all wrong. She sends a young male assistant to fetch very sexy white undies and stockings and she helps me into them.

She decides my breasts do not fit the bra properly, so she slides her hands over my shoulders and lifts them into my bra. At this point, the male assistant helps me adjust my stockings and from then on there are hands and tongues all over me. Soon we are all on the floor without being able to tell whose hands belong to who. I never actually seem to pay for the dress!

Lela, 35, Pharmacy Technician

My recurring fantasy is making love with two men at once. I would never actually do this in real life, however! I've always found physically strong men a turn-on, such as construction workers, men in the armed forces and paramedics. My husband is still a big turn-on. I prefer older men, preferably ones with neatly trimmed beards and moustaches – like my husband!

This is the fantasy I enjoy the most. I am a secretary in the White House. I am tall and slender with long curly blonde hair and emerald-green eyes. I have a fine, pouty mouth and nice long legs – oh, and neatly trimmed pubic hair. One day the president calls me into his office to 'take a letter'. The situation becomes sexual and he demands I get down on to my hands and knees and perform oral sex on him. While this is happening, he presses a button and in walk two of his security guards. They begin to caress me with their hands, lips and tongues. They remove my clothing except for my thong panties. One of the guards kneels behind me and licks my vagina and anus. The other demands oral sex so I'm now forced to give oral sex to both the president and the guard.

Once I am lubricated, the guard behind me takes me roughly in my vagina. He then stops and I give him oral sex, while the other guard takes my vagina and pumps me until he explodes over my bottom. The president then takes me anally. It is a mixture of pleasure and pain. When he is ready to explode he yells for the guard – who has already come – to hold my head back, and the president explodes on to my face.

The last guard to finish asks the president and the other guard to put me on to my back. He places his cock between my breasts. He gets the president and the other guard to pinch my nipples hard, then he explodes over my breasts, mouth and stomach.

Anita, 33, Housewife/Mother
I have favourite themes and subjects to fantasise about, such as swingers' parties, lesbian sex and brief sexual encounters in everyday situations, e.g. over the kitchen sink or at the supermarket or even at the governors/ PTA meeting! My first sexual hero was Clint Eastwood as 'The Man With No Name' in Spaghetti Westerns – lean and mean! I have always been fascinated by women's underwear and loved imagining wearing flimsy, lacy bras, knickers and suspenders. I also like

porno pictures and videos and erotic stories. As far as people who turn me on go, I find Kevin Costner, Tom Cruise and Susan Sarandon very sexy. I am lucky to have a male penfriend and we swap sexual fantasies and some porn too.

This fantasy is set in the backroom of a pub. The landlord has invited a few of his friends round for a meal. He has asked me and a few other barmaids to be waitresses. Everyone knows that sex is on the menu. I stand to one side of the landlord, Pete, as he finishes his wine. He looks at me and quickly licks his lips. I smile down at him and rest my hands on my thighs. Slowly, right before his eyes, I ease my skirt up the slippery nylon of my stockings. I glance across the table and see one of the guests looking at me as first my stocking tops and then suspender straps come into view. Still my skirt moves upwards until my naked, hairless mound is on view. Pete sighs and leans forwards as I part my thighs. I can feel his tongue beginning to probe gently over and between the delicate pink folds of my sex. It's my turn to sigh with pleasure. I open my blouse and begin to caress my breasts, feeling the nipples harden under my touch and the effect of Pete's tongue curling around my clit.

I look across the table and see one of the guests push back his chair. He's sitting with one of his hands slowly working up and down the engorged shaft of his cock. Jenny, another waitress, stands over him, removing her clothes to reveal her curves. She slips two fingers along her furrow and then wipes her juice over his lips. He catches hold of her waist and she straddles his lap, slowly sinking down over the shiny head of his cock. She smiles as his length disappears into her soft, hot tunnel. Her hands rest on his head as he licks, laps and nips his way over her heavy, dark-nippled breasts. I can feel myself flushing hot with arousal as Jenny begins to raise herself up and down on the man's stiff pole.

Pete manoeuvres me around to the edge of the table and I lie back on its cool surface. My legs are resting over his shoulders. Pete has a full view of my open sex, petals puffy and deep pink, glistening with my juices. He makes me gasp as he presses delicate kisses on my inner thighs and blows his cooling breath over my heated sex. My attention is distracted by the feel of large, warm hands covering my flattened breasts, moulding the soft shapes and brushing over my nipples, making them tingle and tighten harder than ever. The stimulating hands belong to Aaron (one of Pete's friends) and, as I look up at him, I see that his eyes are fixed on the sensitive licking Pete is giving to me.

I can feel my climax beginning to build as Pete takes, between his lips, each of my petals in turn and sucks deeply. I move my hips and his tongue slips over my clit and then downwards, teasing around the entrance of my vagina before dipping in and pressing hard against the yielding walls of my tunnel. At the same time Aaron's mouth comes down hard over mine and his tongue is twisting around, drawing me to a sudden trembling. Pete has stood up and without warning plunges his dark, thickly veined cock into my vagina. The combination of being filled so quickly and forcefully and his weight pressing on to my aching clit drives me to another intense climax.

I can see Sarah (another waitress) on all fours on the floor, her mouth wrapped around the cock of a prone guest who in turn is pleasuring another girl with his mouth. It isn't the arrangement of a threesome which is attracting Aaron, though, or the gentle swaying of Sarah's small creamy white breasts, but the steep curves of her hips and buttocks and the open crevice between the firm orbs of flesh. Aaron takes a bottle of oil from the side dresser and slowly and deliberately anoints his stiff, upwardly angled cock, before kneeling behind Sarah. He begins to caress her back with his oiled hands, his hands spread wide over her buttocks and then his thumbs slip down and settle over her arsehole. Sarah tenses and then eases herself back on to his touch. Aaron moves closer, allowing his slippery cock to run over her juice-soaked quim and then up to join his thumbs at her secret place.

Next he takes the bottle of oil and lets a thin trickle flow down the open crevice to pool and trail over the shiny, dark pink head of his cock. Firmly and deliberately he lets his cock slide up and down the trail of oil until Sarah, sensing the tip of his cock nudging against her tight opening, pushes back on it and draws him into her. Aaron grips her hips and pushes deeper until his cock is completely enclosed and his balls are touching her quim. Aaron begins to draw back slowly and slides back, obviously relishing the tight grip of Sarah's anal muscles around his cock.

Unconsciously I begin to tighten my love muscles around Pete's cock in time with Aaron and Sarah's movements. I feel Pete's fingers dig deep into the flesh of my hips and his movements becoming more urgent and less precise. I turn my gaze to look at him as his eyes close and, with long hard stabs, he spurts his hot seed deep into me. Pete slumps forward over me and I cradles his head against my flushed breasts as our juices begin to seep down along my thighs.

Jean, 40, Nurse

I fantasise at least once a day and like to imagine sex in unusual positions – ones I could not physically do! I love the idea of more than one man massaging me and then making love to me. I also fantasise about being blindfolded or restrained in some way. I used to read mildly suggestive books or the women's pages in my mum's magazines. Occasionally I saw my dad's magazines, too. Books were best, however, as I could use my imagination. I always wear stockings and revealing bras or nighties for my lover. I adore massages. My present lover is younger, has ultra-short hair and glasses. He is gentle, kind, and rugged and masterful. He is also full of ideas and even his voice can turn me on.

My favourite fantasy is set in a gym. I am a lot slimmer than I am now. (I have had five children!) I discover that it is Men Only night. They insist, however, that I stay and show me the best use for each piece of equipment. Then I have to savour the delights of sex in the pool and sex in a darkened sauna – clothes and inhibitions totally forgotten.

Betty, 66, Retired Swimming Teacher
I have a recurring fantasy involving being in a hut with lots of other women and men. The men are mostly black and they have lots of different ways of having sex. Needless to say, I am the one selected to go into the chief's room. I used to find films and items of clothing sexy, particularly black lacy items.

Jasmine, 52, Housewife/Home Care Assistant
I fantasise about once a day and each fantasy is different. I enjoy the idea of being secretly watched while being gently fucked. I used to get excited by blue films and my boyfriend exposing himself and wanking in front of me. The first book to turn me on was *No Orchids for Miss Blandish*. Also, turning men on turned me on. These days, seeing the outline of a man's penis through his trousers when he isn't looking is very erotic. Having my bottom pinched by anyone but strangers is also a turn-on.

Being pushed into a large room that is in complete darkness, where there are at least six men and six women all feeling, touching, undressing, stroking and passing on to discover more kissing, licking and probing, is a favourite scene I like to imagine. This scene develops in many different ways from sudden orgasm to double-entry sex and lesbian experiences.

Amanda, 17, Student

I fantasise on average a few times a week. I like the idea of being caught with another woman or being caught masturbating. My current favourite is set in my bedroom with another woman. We are only talking, then we start kissing. By now we have ripped each other's clothes off and are now masturbating each other. She then handcuffs me to the bed. I am powerless to move as she sits on my face while stimulating my clitoris with her tongue. She rolls me over and runs her tongue between my arse cheeks to make the entrance slippery. She then produces a vibrator and pushes it hard into my anus. In the background, I hear a door slam shut, but I ignore it because I am having too much fun. I scream some more and my boyfriend enters the room. We both stare at him, but then we carry on. He joins in. We tie him up. I ride him, while the woman sits on his face. We change positions a few times. It ends when we all come and scream together.

Cassandra, 19, Photographer

My recurring fantasies tend to revolve around such themes as anal sex, doggy-style sex, men in control and force used against me. I used to play 'doctors and nurses' as a child and enjoyed playing the patient. I would be examined intimately by a boy who was playing the doctor. I also enjoyed playing 'mummies and daddies'. I would play the baby, who needed her nappy changed by the boy who played my father. Another turn-on was reading a book written for children, explaining the facts of life with coloured pictures. These days, I like to pretend that I am a naive, inexperienced virgin who knows nothing about sex or foreplay. I have to be taught by a man who knows exactly how to turn on a woman. I love being told that I'm a naughty girl and need to be punished. The punishment must contain some kind of sexual act and I need to be constantly reminded that I'm a very bad girl.

Here is my favourite fantasy. I've just finished travelling around Europe and I've written a book about my adventures on my travels, including my sexual activities. I've made an appointment for dinner with a publisher recommended to me. He has agreed to pick me up from home, instead of meeting in a restaurant. To my amazement he turns up in a chauffeur-driven limousine. I climb in the back, dressed quite professionally. This is the first time we have met as the appointment was arranged over the phone. He is very attractive and looks like Antonio Banderas. There is an instant attraction between us, which we are both aware of. He compliments me on my looks and says that I'm taking a bit of a chance, going out with a strange man I have never met before. Anything could happen.

At this, he kneels down in front of me. I'm a bit shocked but he tells me not to worry or be scared. We don't have to do anything I don't want to do. He just wants to get to know me better. With that he pulls off my blazer and opens my blouse. I have no bra on. He starts to caress my breasts and licks and sucks my nipples. My legs are open now and he pushes up my skirt so it's near my waist. I push off my shoes to make myself more comfortable. He crouches down between my thighs. I have no panties on and he starts to lick at my clitoris, then lower to my vagina opening. He then puts my legs over his shoulders, goes even lower and licks me from my anus to my clitoris and back again. He instructs me to turn over and kneel against the seat, so my breasts are brushing the seat cover. He is right behind me. I watch him put on a condom and take a small tub from his pocket. He smears a lubricant over my privates and anus and also over his cock. He shoves his cock up my arsehole and rubs my clitoris with his fingers.

The limousine suddenly comes to a halt. The door opens and another gentleman steps in. My publisher moves to sit on the seat opposite the other gentleman and instructs me to sit back on his cock, so that it is back inside my arsehole. He then introduces me to the man opposite us, who is called Scott and who looks like Michael J Fox. While I am riding my publisher, Scott leans towards me and kisses me, starting at my mouth, my breasts, my stomach, all the while working his way down. He starts to unbutton his flies and pull out his penis. He starts to masturbate while licking and kissing me. Scott then lies down on the limousine floor, on his back. My publisher instructs me to sit on him and lay my body flat over him, so his cock is in my cunt. My publisher comes from behind, parts my arse cheeks and shoves his cock up my anus again. I am now having two men at once. This is when I usually have an orgasm.

Deborah, 49, Play Officer
When I was fourteen just reading about or seeing a passionate kiss on TV would get me hot and bothered without knowing why. At fifteen I started seeing my first boyfriend. He had a thing about my neck; stroking it, kissing it. At the time it frightened me to death or so I thought. Was I wrong ... He does it now and I definitely know it's not fright I'm feeling! Sometimes, rarely, I have my neck massaged by my boss's boss. It always takes place when someone else is there but I let my mind wander to what might happen if we were alone and not at work.

My favourite fantasy is centred on group sex: two men and one woman. I set the scene in a room, garden or pool. All three are naked; the men are kissing and touching the woman. She is enjoying their caresses but wants to see the men kissing and touching each other. She guides their hands and shows them what she wants them to do. At first they are reluctant but to please her they allow it to continue. They start to relax and find they are enjoying it as well. Touching each other while they are being watched and stroked by a woman really starts to turn them on, which makes the woman hot as well. Group penetration takes place in a variety of positions, leaving everyone gasping. Embarrassment quickly follows, but you know that given the opportunity it will all happen again.

Pamela, 35, Unemployed

I fantasise on average once a day and like to imagine such situations as mutual masturbation and bondage. My partner and I get very turned on by the situations in Black Lace books. Within 30 minutes of reading them my partner has an erection and has to put it to use. I like wearing black leather biker gear. It makes me horny. Gypsies are a particular turn-on, especially the one I am in a relationship with at the moment. He's very rough and ready. When he wants sex, he takes you no matter what and he loves it if you put up a bit of a fight.

I like to fantasise about having sex with three men at once: one having me from behind, one having him from behind and the third standing in front of me, so I can suck him off at the same time.

Opal, 43, Housewife

Although my fantasies are different, the man or men involved are always dominant. They always know what I want and need and always supply it. Until I met my husband, when I was 22, I was totally unaware of my sexuality. I was probably a late developer and, although I had plenty of boyfriends, I barely tolerated their kisses. Having met my husband, I discovered the joy of sex; everything from different and more interesting uses for double cream to 69s. I love sharing a bath or shower and get very turned on by a neat, tight bum. I enjoy reading erotic novels, especially Black Lace ones. I get horny wearing provocative underwear, such as sheer nylon hold-ups. I love the feel of silk or *crêpe de Chine*, especially if I'm wearing nothing underneath.

My favourite fantasy goes like this: I have a terrific job working in a large, beautiful house. Alex, my boss, is an ordinary sort of guy: mid-forties, good firm body, nice looks and the most beautiful eyes – dark and serious. From the very beginning there is a feeling of instant understanding, as if we've always known each other. There is no awkwardness and we talk intimately about ourselves. At the end of my second week Alex tells me how he enjoys fantasies and acting them out.

'Would you consider joining me in my fantasies?' he asks. 'I promise they will not endanger your marriage. It will be for us to enjoy during working hours only.'

How could I refuse, especially as I have a few fantasies of my own I should like to try.

'Yes, I would like that, providing that you never physically harm me. What had you in mind?'

'Since your interview, I've had visions of you standing naked before me. You kneel in front of me and take me into your mouth.'

My hands move towards my jacket.

'No, don't move, because I have since enlarged that scene.' He leans over his desk and presses a buzzer. A moment later the door opens and David, the chauffeur, enters.

'Come in, David. Remove Marie's clothes.'

Slowly David unbuttons my jacket and slips it off, then my skirt, leaving me standing in my black lace bra and pants and sheer nylon hold-ups. My eyes are fixed on Alex. I feel no embarrassment as I know my figure is still good – not as firm as it was, but not flabby. Once I am completely naked Alex reaches out to slide his hands over my breasts, pinching my nipples until they are erect. His hands continue down my body, his nails gently grazing my belly until they reach my pubic hair. His fingers pull at the hair and then one finger slides between my lips.

'I can feel that you are enjoying this; you are already very wet.'

His hands move around to my buttocks where he squeezes them, his fingernails scratching my private opening. I can feel the excitement mounting low in my stomach; a delicious feeling, so warm and so wet.

'Unzip my trousers. Free my penis,' he orders. My fingers are sure as they first open the hook at his waist and then slowly lower the zip. Without being told, I slip my hands inside and push his trousers and pants past his hips. From behind David takes hold of my arms and pulls me back. Alex sits in the armchair, his penis standing proud and his legs wide in front of him. I feel David guiding me towards the chair. He presses me down to my knees. Alex takes my head in both hands and pulls me towards his waiting penis. For a second I resist but then, licking my suddenly dry lips, I reach out for him.

I'm so taken up with my quest, I fail to notice the look that passes between Alex and David. Alex's hands hold my head firmly as he slowly probes my mouth with his penis. Unnoticed, David has removed his clothes and stands to one side of me, a whip in his hand. Alex's knees grip my waist as the whip stings my buttocks.

'Pleasure me as we pleasure you. Relax, feel the whip as it kisses your cheeks. Look beyond the sting, feel the pleasure as it moves over your body,' Alex whispers.

My tongue slides over his penis, and I suck in a strong rhythm as Alex's cock nudges my throat. I can feel the whip as it stings my cheeks ten times. Then hands are kneading my arse, separating my buttocks. A finger is probing my secret opening, which is wet with my own juices. My muscles tense against any further intrusion. A sharp slap relaxes me and then I can feel David's penis as it pushes through the opening.

Now I have two men thrusting into me, faster and faster. My whole mind is swallowed up with feeling. I suck harder as I feel Alex's penis begin to throb, my fingers massaging his balls. A hand reaches around me and I feel David working on my clit, rubbing and pinching until I feel my muscles contract in readiness for my climax. Suddenly my body is swamped with feeling as Alex pumps his come down my throat. David pulls out of my arse and pumps his fluid over my still-stinging buttocks, rubbing it in as if it were a soothing ointment. My own powerful climax breaks and my body trembles. Slowly Alex lifts my face and kisses my lips, his tongue licking his semen that has spilled on to my lips.

'David, the champagne. Let's drink a toast to the future and fantasies yet to be realised.' As I raise my glass with the two men who had just given me such pleasure, I hope I won't have to wait too long for the next time.

Justine, 38, Housewife/Artist

I have recurring fantasies of powerful men, often Arab or Persian. The settings are sunny and sandy, often featuring beautiful tents where I am being held captive. I was nine or ten when I first started to enjoy the attentions my mother's friends paid me. 'Uncle Geoff' was in his late 50s and used to take me golfing with him. I would pull the trolley. He had a bright yellow

E-type Jaguar with soft leather upholstery that wrapped itself around me like an animal. He was slow, deliberate and totally inscrutable. His gentle ministrations seemed always to be offered more as a reward than to satisfy any need on his part.

These days, I get turned on by a calm, slow voice, suggestive of confident control. The smell of leather and clean male bodies too. A smile when it is rare and affectionately bestowed is erotic and I can get horny from a simple fleeting touch on the back of the neck or a steady guiding hand on the elbow in a crowded room. I like men not normally younger than 50. There is no upper age limit.

My favourite fantasy is set in an unfamiliar multi-storey car park. I am looking for my car and become aware of a large, silver limousine creeping along behind me. I stand to the side so it can pass more easily. Instead it pulls up beside me and a young man in a chauffeur's uniform gets out and, grasping my arm, firmly guides me into the back seat, where I am positioned between two middle-aged men in Arab dress. The car has smoked glass at the back and my companions communicate in a language I cannot understand.

As we leave the car park and the vehicle begins to pick up speed, I start to panic. I think of my everyday responsibilities and my car left behind. I lunge across the lap of the man on my left, intent on trying the door. Both men pull me back into position and the man on my right slides his left arm across my back and grasps my left shoulder firmly. Then with his right hand he turns my face towards his face. It is the first time I have looked at him directly and I find myself studying the pock marks and wrinkles on his tanned skin. I hardly dare to look into his deep-brown eyes. His hand slides slowly from my shoulder to the back of my neck and, as he speaks, slowly and quietly, I can feel the tingle of gentle caresses at the top of my spine. Although I cannot understand a word he is saying to me, I'm mesmerised by the sound of his voice. My body feels calm and warm, and at first I'm only vaguely aware that the other man has begun to undress me. My limbs unconsciously assist him while the first man's foreign words eddy and flow over my subconscious. His hands, now cupping my head, move slowly. Long fingers trace the backs of my ears and down along my jaw line. I gaze in fascination at the creamy gradations of the whites of his eyes as I feel my bra slip away from my naked breasts. I long to experience his skilled fingers on my straining nipples.

The car pulls up suddenly and I find myself flung into the large well between the front and back seat. The back of my head is against the driver's seat and my trousers are around my knees. I feel acutely embarrassed and look frantically around for my clothes or something to cover myself with. I can see neither. The man who had until then been quietly undressing me now speaks sharply to the driver. There is an exchange of words lasting several minutes, while I crouch in the recess and peruse my captors. The one with the mesmerising voice is quite tall, folded into the large car. His feet almost reach me, despite the opulent design of the vehicle. The other man is large and barrel-chested with chubby hands and a double chin.

The driver starts to speak in English. 'Your master would like you to know you are not in danger. Would you please to remove the rest of your clothes.' I glance from one man to the other. The fat one is grinning and nodding enthusiastically, while the other simply holds out a large open hand to me. The car is moving quickly now and, as I glance up through the windows, a motorway bridge passes overhead. I reach out and clasp the proffered hand, which enfolds my hand securely, allowing me the balance necessary to remove my remaining garments to the obvious delight of my rotund companion. There is a strong blast of fresh air as my clothes disappear through the fat man's window. I feel extremely vulnerable kneeling in front of the two men, who are still fully clothed.

At this point my fantasy can go in a number of directions, depending on my mood. Sometimes the fat man – his face alight with pleasure – proudly exposes the largest penis I have ever seen, and I position myself between his knees and wrap my lips around its salty tip as his plump hands eagerly fondle my full breasts. Another version has the tall man bend forward and lift my chin once more with his left hand. He draws me towards him, his voice quietly persistent, while his companion ties my hands behind my back and places a blindfold over my eyes. Then a large sheet is thrown over me and secured in place by a collar around my neck. I hear a click as a lead is attached to the collar and I feel the men's hands guide me back on to the seat between them. We travel for some time in silence. I'm aware of the warmth of the men's bodies on either side of me and of my own barely concealed nakedness under the thin sheet. A short plump hand eases its way under the covering and smooths along over my thigh, my skin tingling with anticipation.

Then, as the car turns the corner, my legs open slightly to maintain my balance and a large, chubby finger slips down the crevice below my mons pubis, sending shivers across my abdomen. I no longer want to hold my legs together. I can feel the fat man's hand brushing tantalisingly close to those parts of me that have begun to melt and I wonder if he can feel my dampness. Then the hand is withdrawn and the car begins to slow down. I can hear the clattering hum of a cattle grid as the car passes over it. The voices of all three men speak in turn and I feel small tugs on the collar at my neck. The variety of possibilities, when I reach this point, are almost endless and I have played through many in my mind. The story always ends however, in a beautiful tent in a desert; bright colours, rich smells and heaps of downy cushions all with gold tassels, and a great many well-endowed men clutching and fondling, teasing and penetrating me while the tall, craggy-faced man sits back and controls proceedings omnipotently.

Antonia, 25, Housewife/Mother
I like to fantasise several times a day and have some recurring themes, such as doing it with certain TV stars or being taken at once by my favourite men. Libraries are also a turn-on. My father used to keep quite graphic porno magazines. When I was about ten years old I would creep into his room to read them. They really turned me on, especially because they showed men with hard-ons shafting women in different scenarios. I wish they still produced them. These days, I still like looking at men's dicks – erect ones, particularly. I read explicit material like Black Lace books, too.

My favourite fantasy is set in a library. It is deserted and I'm looking for the romance titles. All of a sudden I hear the door click and I realise I'm alone. I look round from shelf to shelf. Then these three men appear. They are well-known stars of a TV series and they ask me if I can help them. Agreeing, I step up on to a ladder, stretching to the top shelf. I am showing my silk panties. I feel someone's hand run up my thigh, past my suspenders and up to my clit. They part the material and then slip off my silk panties, replacing their hand with their tongue. One of them laps me and sucks me.

I fall off the ladder, only to be caught by another man. The men are all naked with huge stiffies. However, they don't want me to please them, they want to please me. They all fall on to me, removing my clothes and kissing and sucking my breasts and clit, etc. Then each one takes me: one up my cunt, the other up my arse, and one in my mouth. We rock together until I come, then they swap places. After each one has had a turn, they lie there on the floor, caressing me, kissing me and sucking their juices out of me.

Claudia, 40, Musician
Since I am celibate at the moment, my fantasies consist mainly of things I miss a partner doing to me. I love having my breasts licked and sucked, preferably both simultaneously; also having someone go down on me or being fucked awake very gently. I imagine I have two partners; gender non-specific. I used to read a lot of Anaïs Nin and still do. I love the combination of luxury and sensuality and her recognition that eroticism involves the senses.

These days I can even get aroused by *Star Trek* fiction if it is well written. Books where bisexuality is the norm and where polygamy is taken for granted are a turn-on. I'm still aroused by personalities. What happens in your head harms nobody provided it stays there.

Anyway, my favourite fantasy: I'm a guest in a villa where there is a husband and wife in their 40s, a daughter of 20 who is gay and three sons aged 16, 18 and 23. The middle one is also gay and has relationships with his brothers. I walk through the villa opening doors to see who I meet. The possibilities are endless and I never know who I'll meet until I'm there, so to speak. It sounds very clinical written down!

Elaine, 19, Unemployed
I fantasise several times a day and each fantasy is very different. I have always loved the idea/practice of sex doggy-style and of being tied down and ravaged. I like visiting sex shops, too. Porn magazines get me horny.

My boyfriend and I are open about everything and enjoy bringing each other to climax while looking at the magazines.

My favourite fantasy of the moment is set in a health club with my boyfriend. We are in the jacuzzi, relaxing. I'm wearing a very low-cut swimsuit that reveals my slippery breasts. We start to feel very naughty, knowing we're all alone. My boyfriend's hand slips beneath the bubbling water and quickly finds its way to my eager pussy. I slip my fingers around his cock, which is already standing to attention. A guy walks into the room, looking straight at us. To my surprise, my boyfriend continues and motions for the guy to join us. He kneels at the tub and, with encouragement from my boyfriend, I slip him into my mouth. After a few minutes we lay some towels down on the floor and I climb on top of my boyfriend, slipping him inside me slowly. I continue to suck hard on the guy's cock as I'm riding my guy. I feel a cock nudge my bum, then it is thrust deep inside.

I feel delicious, with cocks filling me everywhere. I can't help myself from coming. At the same time, I feel my boyfriend shoot his load. The guy in my mouth serves me a hot, smooth portion and I eagerly take it all, loving every second!

Dec, 31, Housewife

I fantasise about threesomes and rape scenes regularly. I also get off on plenty of foreplay fantasies. When I was younger I used to watch porno films with my friend and we would lick each other until we came. If I slept at her house, she would go underneath the bed covers and I would wake up to her licking me like mad. She would also lick my knickers in front of me. My favourite fantasy is about three or four men stripping me. They force sex on me and one of them licks me while I suck the other. Then the two of them have

77

intercourse, front and back. I am forced to suck another man until he comes and I carry on sucking and swallowing until the man who fucks me front-ways, pulls out of me and makes me suck off my own juices. Then I suck until he comes while I am being fucked backward. That really turns me on! Also I dream of an old man licking me for ages and opening me wide. I open my legs while I watch him lick at my hole and my bum and lap all my come up. He also sucks the wee from my clit. Disgusting, eh? My husband and I have made several films which are very explicit and rude and are a real turn-on.

Cathy, 21, Student
I like fantasising about submissive women and dominant men or experiencing sex with another woman. Being with my husband and another woman at the same time is also a favourite, along with giving my husband oral sex, perhaps with another woman. I love being dominated. In reality, I absolutely hate lecherous men and consider myself a feminist. Sexually I get turned on by the opposite of that; I adore the thought of screwing a middle-aged businessman to give him a thrill, especially if he was aggressive. I love the thought of being at school again and being screwed by a group of male teachers or date-raped (but not hurt). In fantasy land, I'd like a man to piss on me in the shower and slap my tits a bit!

This one is very much a fantasy, as in reality my husband is very gentle, loving, selfless and wouldn't ever hurt me, or anyone. I would love him to be at work one day, when I have a day off from college. I would previously have arranged for a gorgeous girl – maybe an acquaintance – to spend the afternoon and night with me as a surprise to my husband. She knocks on the door at 6 p.m. and we are both a bit shy but obviously fancy each other. I invite her in and we drink some wine and relax. I can't help staring at her body; her tits are like mine; big and sexy, but firm. Through her tight white top, I can see her nipples are stiff. We start touching and she squeezes my tits. We've both been flirting for about an hour and I'm really wet (as I am now in reality, just writing about this stuff!). Anyway, it progresses but we don't lick each other's pussies, just our tits. We have a bath together and my husband returns home to find two sexy, soapy, big-titted girls in his bath.

As this is a fantasy he doesn't act shocked and we don't have to explain ourselves. Instead, he gets out his gorgeous cock and rubs it until he spurts all over our faces and tits. We spend the whole night being his whores – sucking him off and fucking him and each other with courgettes, carrots, etc. We photograph each other in really filthy positions. We are fucked in the arse and slapped by him until he is satisfied.

Anon, 39, Occupation Unknown
I have recurring fantasies about total submission or domination, depending on my mood. I also like to read explicit sex scenes in sexy books and am still discovering things I really like but would never have thought of myself. Group sex with strangers is a favourite fantasy, along with anal intercourse. I get very turned on by nudity. Sexy leather and lace clothing arouses me. I also enjoy fantasising about sex in different places: the park, by a river and in a barn, etc., or sex where there is a risk of being caught.

My favourite fantasy takes place at work. I'm behind my desk with no panties on and there is someone – either a man or a woman – playing with my pussy. Oral sex and sex with a dildo takes place. The perpetrator is hidden by my desk. I move on to a board meeting with both men and women, which turns into a private group orgy. Scenes take place where I end up bound to a chair with people being brought to me and they do anything they like to my body. I am then moved to the boardroom table and have someone's dick in my mouth while someone else plays with and sucks my boobs. Someone gives me oral stimulation and someone else plays with my vagina and anus. I am still tied to the table, so I cannot stop them doing what they want to me.

Megan, 26, Restaurant Helper
I tend to fantasise a few times a week and each fantasy is very different. One of my current favourites takes place in a barn. I walk in and there he is, mucking out hay without a shirt on. I stand and watch him for a moment, then walk over to him and tap him on the shoulder. He turns and is surprised to see me. I am the 'good girl'. I give him my best smile and then pull his face towards mine for a hot kiss. He looks incredulous, but then we strip and I take his huge dick in my hands and he closes his eyes, still not believing it's me. I drop to my knees and take his huge dick into my mouth, enjoying every moment. He spills his seed into my mouth and I suck every last drop. He pulls me up, turns me around and I grab the railing as he fucks me from behind. At that moment a woman walks over to us. I don't know when or where she came from, but the more the merrier.

After we both come, he pulls out and the other woman takes his dick and sucks him as I eat her pussy. After a while he lays the woman down and fucks her as I sit on top of her and she sucks my pussy until we are all satisfied. I have another favourite. It's about a guy at work. We're working together. He's a waiter and I work in the kitchen. I go out and see him. I just have to have him and it can't wait until after work. I grab him and pull him to the ladies' bathroom. Once inside, I undo his jeans, pull them off along with his underwear and then take his huge cock in my hands, then in my mouth. I suck him until he's dry. I then take off my shorts and panties, push him on to the toilet seat and stick his cock into my cunt. He takes my breasts in his hands. As I move up and down on his wonderful cock, we come together. Just as we are both lost in the passion, a customer walks in on us.

Chapter Four
Gender Play

Zeus came as an eagle to godlike Ganymede, as a
swan came he to the fair-haired mother of Helen.
So there is no comparison between the two things:
one person likes one, another likes the other: I like
both.

Greek Anthology, trans. WR Paton
(Cambridge, Mass., 1918)

*T*he Kinsey report of the 1950s declared that all
human beings exist on varying points between
homosexual and heterosexual. In a post-*Ellen* world,
where gay and lesbian programmes frequently feature
on television, and where it's increasingly common for
celebrities to comfortably come out, everything is
neatly categorised. We now have distinct boundaries
of gay and straight – with the occasional anomalous
category of 'bisexual'. Everyone fits tidily in their own
particular box and, as we head towards becoming a
more tolerant society, being gay becomes more socially
acceptable. Right? Well no, actually. Homosexuality

isn't as shocking as it used to be, but prejudice is alive and well.

Partly in reaction to bigotry, many self-labelled gays and heterosexuals have embraced the theory that there is a gay gene – that our sexuality is biologically determined. But what if you have 'confusing' lesbian fantasies and still classify yourself as heterosexual? These days, both psychologists and advice columnists assure worried readers that 'many people have homosexual fantasies, but it doesn't mean you're gay'. In language reminiscent of Victorian psychology, 'confused' straights are told that they're still 'normal' – as long as they recognise it's a phase.

The fantasies detailed here are interesting in two ways: they challenge the culture of heterosexuality, and they point to a 'worrying' bisexual fluctuation in society as a whole. Most of the contributors in this section do not identify as lesbian ('I'm not lesbian, but . . .'), internalising society's fear of bisexuality.

As Black Lace books are aimed towards heterosexual women, it is no surprise that the majority of responses were from women who identify as heterosexual. Despite the growing acceptance of same-sex love, most of the contributors in this section are still entering radical new territory – they're daring to question the culture in which they've been brought up. They're also challenging the biggest social category in our lives, that of sexual orientation, because they're fancying someone different from whom they've been told their whole lives that they should be fancying: men, if you're a woman; women, if you're a man. While it's not particularly radical for self-identified lesbians to have lesbian fantasies, it *is* radical for heterosexual women to admit to similar feelings.

The fact is, we are socialised to be heterosexual from birth. From an early age, especially as women, we are taught to see ourselves in male–female sexual and social pairings – the 'natural' conclusion of which is marriage. Whether or not heterosexuality is a choice is rarely questioned in the way homosexuality's naissance is questioned – because it's a state that has been conditioned into our culture to such an extent that it seems 'natural', as opposed to an 'option'.

As Kenneth MacKinnon puts it in the anthology *Pleasure Principles*, 'Such categorisation involving heterosexual/homosexual and gay/straight, inevitably helps to produce 'reality'. If individuals are socialised through their upbringing in cultures which habitually separate sexualities, which habitually promote one form of sexuality and stigmatise another, then they will internalise to a profound extent the dichotomy in social attitudes. In so doing, they make the dichotomy 'real' even if at one point in history it might not have been so.'[1]

In some ways being bisexual is more of a threat to the status quo than homosexuality, because the lines become blurred. Rather than having a distinct category from which one can easily detach oneself ('Well, I'm obviously not gay – I still fancy men'), suddenly we're sleeping with the 'enemy' – or we may even be the 'enemy' ourselves.

When the strict coding of heterosexual/homosexual can't be controlled, bisexual behaviour becomes 'insidious', 'indecisive', 'promiscuous'. When women, in particular, define themselves outside of traditional sexual prescriptions, they are defining themselves as sexually independent. And, as I've previously mentioned, a sexually independent woman can be a threatening concept to unreconstructed traditionalists of both genders, who make efforts to 'rein in' lesbian sexuality. On the one hand heterosexual men have come to expect non-threatening images of 'girl-on-girl' action, where made-up glossy-haired glamour models gently fondle each other. At the other extreme, the feminist separatist movement has been very disapproving of lesbians making what they see as concessions to patriarchy, such as wearing make-up or admitting to enjoying penetrative sex – even if it's from a strap-on. Both views seem to be sanitised and limited. The reality, as ever, is more diverse than we are led to believe from the stereotypes. The increasing prominence of a fun-loving lesbian culture, where being worthy and political is only as important as clubbing and having fun, is injecting a much-needed dash of colour and humour on to the scene.

The women in this section stake their claim to their own pleasure, and the sexual descriptions are no less explicit than in heterosexual fantasies. There is no reason why they should be. Many people criticise female-generated porn as reading 'as if a man has written it'. The reductive assumption is that women are going to write about sex in a way that's softer and more romantic. As one ad campaign for bras in the 1980s proclaimed: 'Underneath they're all loveable.'

Why do we assume that women identify only with the female characters in narrative? Perhaps sometimes it's really Julia Roberts we want to be kissing in *Pretty Woman*, and not Richard Gere. Who knows – maybe we're fantasising, as Jill does in the Transgender section of this Chapter, that the female lead is our dragged-up boyfriend and *we're* dressed up as the man. The point is that the imagination can't easily be controlled. The power of these fantasies is that they cross gender and sexual boundaries. The two transgender entries even *play* with these boundaries, revelling in turning our strict categories topsy-turvy. There's also Karina, who enjoys voyeuristic man-to-man fantasies; this type of fantasy shows no small debt to the ground-breaking homoerotic work of female writers such as Anne Rice and Mary Renault.

Regarding fantasy across gender lines, MacKinnon

puts a new spin on our old bugbear, Freud, and finds Sigmund has a surprisingly positive outlook: 'Freud might argue unregenerately that the female spectator receives masochistic pleasure in beholding her passivity. More interestingly, his work on fantasy suggests that the subject's relation to fantasy is constantly shifting and that we cannot predict from knowledge of the subject's gender, class or social positioning, for example, what sites of identification he or she will occupy in relation to the scenario of fantasy.[2]

Two of the women in this section mention the need to have a man finishing them off after they've played around with a woman for a while; this is also a common straight male fantasy – that a woman, at the end of the day, needs a real-life cock to do the job. But with scenarios that involve transvestism, strap-on dildos and hermaphrodites, nothing is too predictable. The stories have a heavy emphasis on pleasure and a low emphasis on shame. What's more, they point to the fact that our convenient sexual-orientation boxes of gay, straight and bisexual may be putting limits on our changing – more fluid – sexualities.

Women With Women

Kefia, 29, Cosmetics Rep.
I fantasise a few times a week and have recurring themes. They are of being seduced when innocent but curious by an older woman, or of sucking off a very large, hard and often black cock. I used to enjoy thoughts of being caressed and kissed and of exploring a partner's body and giving each other much pleasure. Female bodies were always more attractive, but I was also fascinated by a cock getting harder and bigger.

These days, during love-making, I like having a partner use words which would in other circumstances be objectionable, and I want to feel comfortable enough to use them also. I also enjoy the idea of a male lover talking me through masturbation over the telephone. When having coffee or a meal out, I like to observe women of my age or slightly older, or more mature men, and to fantasise about them!

My current fantasy goes like this: I'm around 23 years of age and have had no relationship with someone of my own sex since my schooldays, being shy, and my previous dates with boys having been disappointing or worse. I begin to have thoughts of sex with a girl around my age.

As a result of placing an ad in the personal column of a newspaper, I start corresponding with a girl. The photo she sends further attracts me. She is unashamedly lesbian, she writes. Her letters contain little more than hints of a sexual nature. As we get to know each other, her letters and photo help stimulate me to play with myself, and I always come fairly quickly. Before long we arrange to speak on the phone, and when I call her, her voice also turns me on. She tells me how she is longing to meet me and how she likes to make love. Then she tells me that just talking about it is making her wet and making her want to masturbate. I admit I'm feeling the same way and she tells me she wants to hear me getting worked up and masturbating until I come.

I am really worked up by now and begin to masturbate while she tells me to imagine what she is doing to me. She is very descriptive. As I get closer I can hear her little moans. Very soon I come and, almost at the same time, I hear her crying out that she is coming, too. We arrange to meet soon after that. She is to stay at my flat for the weekend and, getting ready to meet her, I'm nervous and a little embarrassed at facing her after our graphic telephone conversations. But I'm also excited at the thought of being with her and having her make love to me.

When we meet, we are comfortable with each other and, during a meal before going home, I feel more and more turned on by her presence. I have a mad thought that I wish she would touch me right there in public as we sit close, without, of course, anyone else being aware of it. But she doesn't, and we go to my flat. As soon as we are inside, we embrace. She gives me a deep kiss that gets me going. Her hand wanders over my bottom and her fingers slide down the crevice between my buttocks. She then tells me she had planned to play it more calmly but she wants me, and we go into the bedroom and undress. She is darker than I and has a thick cluster of pubic hair. In bed she at once begins to kiss me, starting on my lips, down to my breasts briefly, brushing down my body and equally briefly nuzzling into my pubic hair.

I am really turned on by now and she returns to my breasts to lick and suck the nipples until they are standing hard. I feel so hot between my legs. Caressing and kissing me, she lowers herself to my thighs and gently parts them, kissing the inside of my thigh and gradually going up to my wet opening pussy.

My face is burning and I'm aching to have her make love to me for hours. She starts to lick me slowly and gently, eventually going up to my clit, easing it out of the folds and sucking gently. She licks it over and around and I feel myself close to orgasm. She must know it because she gets more passionate in her kissing and pushes her face into my pussy. Her tongue brings me closer and closer. I feel I could scream. Then my thighs rear up as I go into an intense orgasm and she continues nuzzling until I am drained.

She lies quietly with me as I come round from the exhausting experience. I can tell she wants to come and I begin to kiss and caress her, hoping I am pleasing her as I am inexperienced. I more or less copy what she did to me. Afterwards she tells me I am a lovely lover and later that night, after a period of wandering about the flat naked and after eating light food and drink, we make love again for hours.

The next night we have our first 69 as well as using a double-ended dildo that she brought with her. Later I'm awakened by her fingers on my pussy, and when she sees that I am awake she nuzzles up to me and starts on my clit. Sleepily, I start wanting it again. That is the start of our relationship together, which doesn't progress much further than that because otherwise it would not be the same fantasy! I will just add that often I indulge this fantasy in more compact form and just as often it does not run its full course. It all depends on how I am feeling before I start.

Clara, 22, Dental Nurse
Lots of my fantasies include myself with another woman. I used to fantasise only about men. I liked to watch sexy films, and I always tried to please my man; I never thought of my own satisfaction. I can now fantasise about women and not feel guilty. I now love reading sexy books rather than watching films.

My favourite fantasy is that I'm working behind the bar in a gay club. This woman asks me if I'm gay. I say, 'No, at least, I don't think I am.' She asks if I've ever slept with a woman and I reply that I haven't. She asks if I would like to go back to her place. I go, and we sit and chat, have a drink and she touches my face. I can't take my eyes off her chest. I notice she is not wearing a bra. She catches me staring. She asks me if I like her boobs. I say, 'Yes.' So she stands up and takes her blouse off, very slowly. I'm so turned on, I can't believe it. She kneels down, leans across and starts unbuttoning my blouse. She takes it off me, then touches me. I'm tingling. She then stands up and pulls me up with her. She takes off her skirt and I take off mine, so that we are both standing there naked. She kisses me and caresses me. Then she leads me to the bedroom. She puts a strap-on dildo on me. We kiss passionately and she gets on top of me and starts riding me. It feels great. I've got a brilliant view of her. I've got my hands on her breasts and she is moaning. I am so turned on watching and touching her while she is coming.

Rosemary, 26, Housewife
A recurring fantasy I have is of my husband and myself having a threesome with a man or woman. I also like to imagine myself having a long-standing relationship with another woman. I used to get aroused by girls getting changed for PE at school, too. These days I like to see my husband wearing a G-string and I perform oral sex on him. I also get turned on by certain women I see or meet. My favourite fantasy involves seeing a woman who shops regularly in my town. After a while we start acknowledging each other. One day I'm in a café, when she comes in. There is nowhere for her to sit, so I invite her to sit with me. We get on really well and exchange telephone numbers. That evening she phones me and says she can't get me out of her mind. I tell her that I feel the same way. We arrange to go back to my house while my husband is at work.

It's summertime and very hot. We are both wearing skimpy shorts and T-shirts. I make her a cold drink while she goes outside in the garden and lights a cigarette. I take out her drink and, as I pass it to her, I trip and the cold drink spills over her lovely round boobs. Her nipples go rock hard instantly. There's a towel on the washing line, so I grab it and start drying her titties. I apologise profusely and tell her to come inside and borrow a T-shirt while I wash and dry her T-shirt and bra. We go upstairs and she removes her top and bra, and I can't help myself. I start caressing her nipples and kissing her. This is the start of a wonderful relationship. Then one day my husband catches us!

Jade, 27, Bakery Assistant
My recurring fantasy theme is of being seduced by my female boss and her female secretary. I also get off on the idea of being a sex slave. Films turned me on at an early age. Later on I started to read erotic books. These days I still watch porn movies to get aroused, especially those with two, three and four women playing with dildos and vibrators. I like reading erotica, particularly Black Lace novels and books by Nancy Friday.

My favourite fantasy takes place in an office. I am an office clerk. The boss is a high-powered woman aged between 45 and 50 (just the age I like my women to be in my fantasies). I didn't think the boss had noticed me over the last six months but, one afternoon, I am told she wants to see me. I have butterflies in my stomach. I go into the boss's office and she is sitting on her desk with her legs crossed. The company I work for sells larger women's underwear. The boss tells me that their regular model is off sick and would I mind modelling some of their products. She shows me some underwear that wouldn't cover a flea. As there is no changing room, my boss says it's OK to get changed in her office.

I start to undress in front of my boss and I can feel my juices starting to flow. I am totally naked when Chris, the boss's secretary, walks in. She tells me that I have got very sexy breasts. I blush. I put on the underwear, which has no crotch, and the bra that has nipple clips attached. My boss suggests taking a few photos of me. She tells me which positions she wants me in. Then she tells me that there are a few things she wants me to try out. Chris brings in a briefcase with vibrators and dildos in it. I am told to get on my hands and knees so Chris can insert a vibrator into my fanny. It feels very big. My boss takes a few shots and then tells me to lie on my back with my legs wide open. She then instructs Chris to put on a strap-on dildo and screw me. I tell her I don't want Chris to do any more things to me. She tells me that if I don't do these things I will lose my job. She tells Chris to fuck me until I beg her to stop. Chris pushes the biggest dildo into me and starts to fuck me and lick me like there's no tomorrow. I come about four times and my boss tells Chris to suck, bite and lick my breasts.

Chris makes me come once more, then she tells me to get on my hands and knees. I do as I'm told. Just as I'm about to ask what is going to happen to me, my boss sticks a vibrator up my arse and I drop to the floor with pain. My boss keeps the vibrator buzzing as she pushes it in and out of my tight arsehole. I am begging her to take it away. She tells me I'm going to be her sex slave and I have to call her Mummy from now on. I'm taken back to my mummy's house, where I'm told to take all my clothes off. I am told from now on that when my mummy comes into the room, I must drop to my hands and knees so that if she wants to, she can either fuck me with a dildo or stick a vibrator into my pussy. I'm told that I must sleep in my mummy's bed and every morning, before we get out of bed, I must give her oral sex and suck her tits for half an hour. She also says that I must let Chris fuck me with the biggest dildo I have ever seen. If I refuse to do anything, my mummy or Chris say that I will have a vibrator pushed up my tight arse.

I get up one morning without giving my mummy oral sex or sucking on her tits. She calls me back into the bedroom and tells me to lie on my stomach and spread my legs. I beg her not to punish me. Chris comes into the bedroom and I run to her and beg her to ask Mummy not to hurt me. Chris puts her arms around me and tells me to suck on her tit like a baby. I do, but as I am sucking on her tit, Mummy pushes a vibrator up my arse and I cry out in pain. Mummy tells me that it is for my own good. Chris tells me to lie down on the bed and she will hold me till the pain goes away. As I'm lying in her arms, she tells Mummy to put a vibrator up my pussy, so that I have vibrators buzzing in every hole. I am crying for them to stop. Mummy puts on a strap-on dildo and so does Chris. They take out the vibrators and Chris lies on the bed. I'm told to sit on her and Chris pulls me on to her. Mummy inserts her dildo up my arse. They both start to fuck me together. I come.

Jacqui, 48, Shop Assistant
I tend to fantasise about sex with another woman or several, and also three- and foursomes. I used to get turned on by wearing silk nightwear. Dancing close with a boyfriend was very erotic and various erotic titles such as *Lady Chatterley's Lover*, *The Pearl*, *The Perfumed Garden* and films such as *Emmanuelle* and *Bilitis* were all favourites. These days I can get turned on by the atmosphere at the right time or even a good drink. A hot summer's day or the right music gets me in the mood.

My favourite fantasy takes place when I am on the way to the supermarket. Just before I go in, two teenage girls stop me and ask if I would help them do something. They go into a small room and I follow. They shut the door and, before I realise it, one of them is before me and one is behind me.

The one behind starts stroking my hair and my back. I can feel her breathing against my neck. I ask her what she thinks she's doing. She says I have nice hair and a lovely neck. She kisses my neck and I try to move away, but the one in front is standing right against me. She says that I have a nice figure and that my nipples

93

look very responsive. She rubs her flat palm across the front of my blouse and I can feel my nipples hurting because they are so hard. Her friend is now kissing my neck, running her tongue from my shoulder up to my ear. The girl in front is gradually undoing my blouse button by button. I seem frozen to the spot. I can't move. She pulls the blouse from my skirt, leaving my stomach naked and only my bra covering me. She pushes her mouth on to mine and starts to kiss me on the lips. I try to stop things but my resistance just doesn't seem to work. I can feel her tongue pushing against my lips and her teeth nipping at the edge of my mouth. Her friend behind me is still kissing around my ears (a weak spot for me), pushing her tongue deep into my ear, making sexy noises. My heart is beating so fast now and I can feel my sex lips peeling open with my wetness.

The girl at the back puts her hands under my blouse and I feel my breasts drop as she unclips my bra. Her hands come around me and she holds my naked breasts from underneath. Her friend takes this opportunity to push her tongue into my mouth and I know I am lost. The girl behind stops touching my breasts and undoes the front of the other girl's top. She has no bra and, when she leans against me, I can feel her hot breasts pushing against mine. The feeling is so sensual that I'm fighting for breath against her tongue in my mouth. The zip on my skirt is being pulled down and my skirt just seems to slip to the floor. I am not wearing a slip, so my panties are all I have on. They are very wet. The girl kissing my mouth stops, and they pull me on to a small table that was in the corner. I am on my back and my breasts and mouth are being kissed with a vengeance. My legs and arms are being held firmly each side of the table. I notice that both girls are now naked, as they rub their bodies against me. The one holding my top half is kissing my breasts and stomach. As she is leaning over me, her sex is right near my mouth. She keeps lifting herself so that the top end of her vagina touches my face.

The other girl keeps touching the edge of my pants and rubs me through them. She doesn't seem to be in as much of a hurry as her friend. Her fingers keep creeping under the leg hole and brushing against my lips. I am getting more and more frustrated and I move about to try to push things along a bit. I start to push my tongue into the other girl's wet vagina. She sighs and I realise that she must have been feeling the same as myself. As I lick her she becomes wetter and wetter and my mind becomes totally absorbed in what I'm doing. I am finding it a beautiful experience. My pants are now being pushed down my legs and the cool air around the top of my legs is calming me slightly. My legs are splayed open and my lips are, too. A warm tongue moves up my thighs and around my openings.

The girl at my sex tells her friend how wet I am, but this girl just murmurs and carries on sucking and pinching my breasts. I can feel my nipples being pulled. They ache with sexual wanting and feel an inch long. My vagina is now so open and wet that my clitoris feels as prominent as my nipples. The girls suck and lick; even my bottom is given the same treatment. I have never experienced this before. I can feel my excitement growing, the more I lick and the more I am licked; it's a vicious circle. I feel fingers inside me. There is no resistance; they go in easily. The girl at my head lets go of my hands so I can pull her on to my face and touch her. She just lets me do what I want to. I suppose she is nearly there, too. My stomach is beginning to knot up with tension and my orgasm is coming to a head. My fingers are now going faster and faster.

The girl I am touching says to her friend that she thinks I'm coming. She in turn touches me harder and deeper. I think she is feeling for my G-spot, but mine isn't easy to find. Then I notice something else. While she's been pushing her fingers deep into me, her little finger has been entering my bottom. I am so wet down there that my bottom is soaked as well. The feeling is not as revolting as I had thought it might be. With her fingers in my vagina and her other fingers deep inside my bottom, my excitement is building up so quickly that when I come I cannot believe it has happened so fast. The liquid is pouring from me, even though the girl is pushing her face right against me, drinking as fast as she can. The girl above me shudders and tenses her vagina. My fingers are gripped by the muscles in her vagina so hard that I can't get them out. Her friend leaves me and goes round to her. She kisses her very hard on the mouth, takes hold of her nipples and squeezes as hard as she can. I feel her muscles relax and I can remove my fingers. Her orgasm is so intense that she screams out loud. Her juice pours on to my hand and I put it to my mouth. The taste is surprisingly inoffensive, unlike what I had always imagined. They help me dress and smarten myself up. They say they hope I don't tell anyone about what just happened. I say that my husband would never believe me if I told him, but that the experience was the thing that fantasies are made of.

Cath, 28, Secretary
I like power and control games in my fantasies. I also like confined spaces and the sea. These things arouse me. When I was younger, many things turned me on, such as stockings, shoes, school teachers, my mother, *Lolita*, *The Stud* and *Venus in Furs*. Tall men and women get me going these days; also powerful or pseudo-powerful people. I like to imagine people in formal, elegant clothes with breathy, sexy voices.

Here is my latest favourite fantasy. I am walking

along in the West End of London, window shopping, when I see a beautiful boutique, full of luxurious lingerie and gorgeous formal business suits. My curiosity aroused, I enter and am asked by the assistant if I would like to try anything on. I select an exquisite set of underwear. The assistant ushers me to a small but beautifully furnished room at the back of the shop and, unexpectedly, three more women appear. The door is locked and I am then taken to another room, which is more like an operating theatre. The four women (all tall and very pretty) then don white coats and tell me they want to turn me into an absolutely gorgeous goddess of a woman. They fasten me to the operating table and, after drugging me, they work swiftly to beautify me. They give me fabulous breasts, a lithe body, long legs and a pouting mouth. My eyes are made bluer, my hair blonder. Even my feet are made sexy.

Then, when I am roused from my slumbers, I am pampered and prettified further. My legs are shaved so they are completely smooth. My eyebrows are plucked and my lashes curled and dyed, so that they feel false. My nails are painted bright red and I am made up perfectly. The women then bring in an array of fabulous underwear. They fit me with a bra that fits like a second skin and slide me into delightfully slinky, silk knickers. I try on lots more: G-strings, bodies and basques, etc. Then I am dressed for business. I am assisted into ultra-sheer stockings and a black suit. I put on a pair of vertiginous stilettos and I go over to a mirror to revel in my new, beautiful self. The women tell me I look gorgeous, and I ask them what I can do to thank them for turning me into a beautiful being. They reply that there is nothing I can do except, if I want to, I could have sex with them. I dither for a while and accept.

We then enter a red bedroom with a four-poster bed.

I am divested of my clothes and led to bed. We take turns to have sex and it gets increasingly more dominating. I am strapped to the bed and aroused by a variety of dildos that they strap on. I lie and kiss for an eternity and then have sex again. A man is brought in and we dominate him, then he arouses me even further. I eventually get bored so I wallow in a bubble bath and I then leave, feeling renewed (but maybe a bit ashamed or guilty as well.)

Wendy, 42, Research Assistant
My fantasies are always of a lesbian nature. Often the subjects are other girls and I am either looking at or compiling a book or film on their actions. I invariably have orgasms at such times. I first started to admire other women's bodies in my early twenties. Prior to that I had been more less hetero and had even been married for a short time. Then a girlfriend showed me a lesbian video and later, slightly drunk, she seduced me. Since then, a woman's body is all I have wanted. I especially like whipping scenes involving only women in my fantasies. I always look out for these in Black Lace books.

I myself love to whip and be whipped by other lovely lesbians. I am about to be whipped shortly by my current girlfriends, both at once – front and rear! My favourite fantasy is set in a girls' college. It is a hotbed of lesbian activities. Early in the morning one of the teachers presents herself at the headmistress's study. Her secretary, before announcing her, admits that the head, called Sandra, is in a very sexy mood. After some kissing and fondling, the teacher is shown in to the head. The teacher, Gloria, has a terrific body with large, firm breasts and a lovely bottom. The head asks for one of the new girls to be sent to her for punishment on any pretext. Sandra wants to make love to this girl. Before the teacher goes, the head demands to be whipped with one of the many canes in the office. Gloria willingly complies and orders Sandra to bend over the whipping stool. She then lifts her skirt and pulls down her panties. The head's bottom is then laid bare and Gloria proceeds with the whipping. She gives about 50 strokes and the head's bottom is striped with angry red weals.

The head, meanwhile, has several noisy orgasms, begging Gloria to whip her harder. She then lays back on an easy chair, opens her legs and commands Gloria to suck her cunt. This brings more mutual orgasms to both women. All this has been seen by Linda, the secretary, through a two-way mirror. Linda is busy masturbating fiercely for several orgasms. Gloria leaves shortly afterwards, saying that she will send up Patsy who, she says, knows all about lesbian love. Patsy arrives and Sandra sternly tells her that she is about to be punished. She meekly agrees and, having removed her skirt and panties, bends over the stool. Sandra admires her lovely bottom, which is enhanced by regulation stockings and suspenders. She then removes her own skirt and allows Patsy to see her freshly whipped cheeks. Patsy is obviously turned on by the sight and waits for her share. Sandra tells her that she will receive eighteen lashes (her age) in groups of six. The whipping starts. The first six are given quickly, marking the soft flesh of Patsy's bum. The next six are given more slowly and Patsy gasps between each stroke. Sandra strokes her burning cheeks with a cool hand and asks whether Patsy has had enough. Patsy begs Sandra to continue and orgasms between each of the last four strokes. Sandra then applies cooling cream to the whipped cheeks, inserting her finger deeply into Patsy's love nest, causing further orgasms. Sandra then kisses Patsy passionately and asks her to call at her house that evening for 'real lesbian lust'. Linda and

Gloria both watch these activities between bouts of their own loving.

Patsy arrives at Sandra's house that evening, in brief, casual clothing. Sandra has a short, transparent negligée on, which emphasises her ample figure. She quickly takes this off and, having undressed Patsy, they admire each other's bodies. Gloria sucks greedily at Patsy's inflamed nipples before moving down to her cunt. She sucks her to orgasm after orgasm and mutual love goes on all night. At this point I am overcome with passion and finger my cunt to glorious orgasms.

Beatrice, 60, Retired
My fantasies usually involve submitting to a dominant female who ends up punishing me. This is at odds with my outward persona (I am not a lesbian) and sex with women is only in my fantasies. I read *Moll Flanders* and, later, *Lady Chatterley's Lover* (underneath the bedclothes at home). I went to a co-ed grammar school and went about in a gang of six; three girls and three boys. We had fun behind the games pavilion. I never went too far, I must say. We didn't in those days. One thing I recall especially is us three girls got hold of a razor from a boy and shaved each other's pussies in a cloakroom. That was a turn-on I've never forgotten. These days, I find being stroked with a feather (unexpectedly and with my eyes closed) a turn-on. I also like to have my nipples sucked and licked and I find being spanked on my bare behind really gets me going. It turns me on terrifically. Seeing a man in tight jeans with a neat bum also arouses me.

My favourite fantasy is about a woman who was a lecturer at college, when I was a student of seventeen. There were one or two incidents then that led me and some of my friends to suspect this woman could have been a dominatrix. Anyway, my fantasies conjure up a woman like her. She is tall, athletic, beautiful and I am in a stable after riding. This woman, who is in charge of the riding lesson, says I am not doing my best. I argue and answer back. She tells me to apologise. I refuse. Then she takes me by the arm and shakes me. I kick out and catch her shin, which provokes the mistress to anger. There is a struggle, and she pushes me over some straw bales and pulls my breeches down to my knees, pinning my legs down. I am wearing a thong so as not to have a panty line, and the mistress is cross about this, adding to the tension.

I know what is going to happen, and I can already feel myself getting wet. The riding crop comes down across my bottom for the first time and I yelp. She tells me that if I yell again, she will whip me an extra cut. I do my best and only cry out once, earning the extra stroke. When the mistress has finished with me she throws down the crop and lies behind me. She kisses me on the buttocks, in my cleft. Then she strokes me with a finger before pushing two fingers into my cleft. She finds my bottom hole and runs a finger round the puckered edge. She scratches the skin with her nail. All the time I am lying there sobbing and the pain in my behind is doing strange things to me. Heat is spreading through me from back to front, and I can tell that I am not far off a come.

Then the mistress intrudes with a hand between my legs and thrusts two fingers up into my sex. I am soaking. She removes her hand and puts her fingers to my lips. She tells me to lick her fingers. 'It's you,' she says. 'Lick it, all of it, lick it all off, taste yourself.' I do this. She then puts fingers into my sex again, up between the lips, which are swollen and engorged by this time. She swivels her fingers around and finds my little bud. It is unbearable. I cannot prevent coming. By putting her other hand to my back cleft and pushing a finger into my bottom hole as far as she can, she brings on my orgasm, a really huge one.

Mandy, 22, Mother/Housewife

I enjoy thinking about two women making it together. One of them must be me. I remember being really turned on by any sex in films. I also saw a friend's magazine with lots of naked women and it really turned me on. These days anything can lead me to fantasise; erotic books especially.

My favourite fantasy is of being tied down or hand-cuffed to a bed by a woman with large breasts, who then explores my body with her tongue, her hands and any object that will fit into my fanny. I try to get out of the handcuffs but she won't let me. She then puts her fanny over my mouth and I can't help but use my tongue on her. She then smacks me across the bottom and starts calling me names, such as 'bitch' and 'slut'. By then, you can guarantee that one of my kids will wake up and my dream has been shattered.

Alison, 22, Mother

I fantasise a few times a week and always about myself and another woman or group of women. When I was in my teens, myself and two friends – one male, one female – went for a walk. We started to play truth or dare. My dare was how long I could last while the boy touched my body. I still had my clothes on. When he started to touch my uncovered skin, my arms, neck and legs, it felt nice because it didn't feel wrong. I love seeing tall men in uniform. My husband is a security guard, and when he is in uniform he looks so sexy. It makes me all wet at the thought of how domineering uniformed men can be.

Here is my favourite fantasy. I go out to a nightclub and I notice a group of women watching me. They follow me to the toilets. When I come out of the cubicle there is only one of them left. The woman grabs my hand and leads me through a door. The room is lit with a red light and there are naked women in groups of two and three. I am taken to the centre of the room, where two women start to strip me slowly and sensually, running their fingers over my skin. The feeling is unbelievable. They start to stroke my nipples to erection, rolling them between their fingers. I start gasping with excitement. One of them starts to kiss my breasts, while the other slowly moves down my body, kissing each part of the skin she comes to. I can feel myself getting wetter, knowing where she is heading. I part my legs willingly. She inserts one finger, then another. Pulling them out, she licks them teasingly. She puts her head between my legs and parts my swollen lips. I'm waiting with desire for the feelings I know so well. Suddenly it's there, her tongue exploring me inside and out. The other women are still sucking my nipples. The pleasure is too much to take. I can't take any more. The warmth spreading through my body is hitting me like an explosion. I orgasm so loudly that I can hear my juices begin to flow. There's a loud applause from the groups of women who have been watching with excitement.

Naomi, 20, Cashier
I have a recurring fantasy about my fiancé catching me with another woman and then joining in with us and her partner. I was about thirteen or fourteen when I first discovered my lower regions. I didn't really know much about it and I was the only virgin in my high school. I'm making up for lost time with my fiancé now! Sex outdoors is a big turn-on, ever since this happened to myself and my partner on the way home from a party.

My favourite fantasy starts with me in the shower, getting ready for a girl's night out. My fiancé has just gone to the shops. I was immensely turned on before he left and now that he is gone, I've taken the shower head off the wall and changed the setting to jet. As I spray the water over my clit, I can feel the start of an orgasm building up. But I hear noises and have to stop.

As I step out of the shower to investigate, I see a strange black girl coming up the stairs. She's wearing a short black skirt with stockings and a suspender belt with a bra top. She isn't the smallest of women. Before I can say anything about her being in my house, she's right up close, smelling my skin. As I am still horny from the shower, I drop my towel and let her do as she pleases. She's got me on the bed with her head buried in my puss. I've been licked out before but never like this. She has such a long tongue that she manages to go deep inside me, filling up my whole puss. I just want her so much that I come, and to my shock she swallows me as I'm coming. I haven't noticed but my fiancé is in the doorway, watching. He yells at her to get out and I start getting dressed. When I hear him coming upstairs, I prepare to get shouted at but, instead, he gives me the best fucking I've ever had.

Jeanette, 55, Taxi Driver
I fantasise several times a day. Usually the scenarios are full of bondage or sex with vibrators. They are usually scenes with women. When I was younger, just a film that showed a bare bum was very sexy. I remember being aroused by Marianne Faithful doing up her leather biker's suit in the 60s movie, *Girl on a Motorcycle*. Low-cut dresses were also very sexy and one of my hottest experiences was my husband shaving my pussy.

My favourite fantasy goes like this. I am taken into a room. There are several women standing around a hospital couch with a post at each corner. My wrists are strapped to the two top posts and my ankles are strapped to the others. The posts are pushed apart and I am exposed for all the women to see. They all put on rubber gloves. They pour oil over my tits and begin to rub it in. They pinch and squeeze my nipples until they become sore. Then two of the women start to nibble my nipples.

The oil is poured over my stomach and then downward. The women start to rub the oil into my cunt and around my arse. They make sure they don't touch my clit. They pull my lips apart and I can feel a very large vibrator being pushed in. I feel another much smaller one being pushed into my arse. Then they rub my clit. As I come, I scream and wet myself.

Carrie, 19, Student
In my fantasies I have recurring themes of domination and rape, or sex with women or a teacher. These are people I know. I used to get very turned on by men's backs. I don't care that much for them now. I do love Latin American men. There is something very sexy about them. I think the hint of sleaziness is what turns me on most. I like watching sex; so far only in films. I need more exhibitionist friends!

The setting for my favourite fantasy is an office. It is a top-floor office overlooking a city. I'm the smart-suit, good-shoes, high-flyer type. There is a new admin worker in the shape of Pamela Anderson on my team. She is known to be sexually naive. After a month of blatant sexual attraction on my behalf, we finally begin to develop an extension to the boss/subordinate relationship. I discover that she had been in numerous abusive relationships with men. Although not homosexual myself, I suggest she try sex with a woman. She is coy and unwilling. But in the dimly lit empty office in the early hours I set about seducing her. She is up against a filing cabinet and I kiss her softly on the lips, gently cupping her breasts. She doesn't know whether to respond and shyly just succumbs, thanks to my sucking those nipples. After fingering her I bend her over a desk, hitch her skirt up, pull her pants down and part her buttocks and work my tongue into her anus. I always come at this point and the fantasy fades.

Men With Men

Karina, 23, Cashier/Food Service

I consider myself bisexual and my fantasies usually revolve around men together. I hope one day to be present while two men are enjoying each other. I have a very varied fantasy life. Some of the people and situations that turn me on are my best woman friend, redhead women and S&M. I also get turned on by contrasting colours; for example, black and white, Nicole Kidman and Brad Pitt, cats, anal and oral sex (I love giving blow jobs and eating pussy), erotic novels and fantasising about anything and everything. Leather still gets me going, and I get a kick out of sexual letters, Black Lace books and reading romance novels; these were forbidden when I was a child. I also like to masturbate to *Penthouse* and *Forum* (the Men With Men section).

Here is my favourite men with men fantasy. I close my eyes and find myself transported to a brick house in the middle of nowhere. I walk up the steps and find the front door open. I walk inside and down a long corridor, following the sound of muffled voices. I see a door left partly open. I look inside and see two men kissing. The older man (Kurt) is tall with blond hair and is about 32. The younger man (Jake) isn't as tall but is also blond, his hair in a crew-cut. He is about 25. They are both very fit but the younger one is thinner.

Kurt starts to undress Jake. He unbuttons his shirt, kissing every inch of his skin. Jake slides his fingers through Kurt's hair and kisses him. Their tongues meet, their mouths collide and Kurt rips Jake's shirt off his body. He clutches his arse to pull Jake closer.

Slipping his hands down Kurt's back, Jake pulls Kurt's shirt from out of his pants and glides his hands up and down Kurt's bare skin. Sliding his hands around to the front, Kurt unsnaps Jake's jeans and slides them down his thighs. Kurt touches Jake's cock with his fingertips and it jumps to attention. Jake moans. Kneeling down, Kurt gently places Jake's cock in his mouth. Jake groans, and plunges his cock down Kurt's throat. In, out, in, out, faster and faster, Jake plunges in until Kurt can barely hold on for the ride. Kurt seizes Jake's arse and, pulling it apart, rams his middle finger into his arsehole. Jake screams in ecstasy, coming in Kurt's mouth.

Before Jake can finish coming, Kurt topples him to the floor and thrusts his cock into Jake's arse. Jake groans. Kurt moans and slides his cock in and out of Jake. In, out, in, out, faster and faster, Kurt fucks Jake, cramming his cock to the hilt into him. There is a look of pure delight on both their faces. Just as I come, I see Kurt and Jake come. Kurt pulls out. They fall to the floor, kissing and holding each other. Suddenly I find myself transported back into my bed and fall asleep. This is one of my favourite fantasies. I even stopped to play with myself during the writing of it.

Anonymous, 39, Occupation Unknown

In a previous marriage I was upset to find that my husband was a transvestite. Initially it was fun and exciting, but I didn't want it as an everyday thing. I had lots of fun taking part in light bondage games and this still excites me. I like anything to do with largeish women. They are so sensual. Nubile girls and boys are totally boring to me. Macho men and large ladies, really sensual people who have experienced life. I think a butch, hairy man can be sexy, as can a large attractive lady. Large breasts and bottoms signify a real woman who enjoys being a woman.

My current fantasy is that my husband and I are staying in a classy hotel. We decide to experiment with a little light bondage. I secure him facedown on the bed with his hands and feet secured to each corner bedpost. What he is slightly freaked out by is that I've raised his bottom on pillows. He likes me to use my finger on his arse, but I have something else in mind. I blindfold him and let him enjoy the sensation of having a vibrator used on him. Then, unknown to my husband, I invite the hotel manager – a very handsome gay man who has often eyed up my husband – to our room. He enters silently and begins to caress my husband, who still thinks it's me doing these things. The manager positions himself behind my husband and pushes his cock inside my husband's arse. What a sight: two sets of balls slapping around side by side! My husband only discovers what's going on when the manager lets out an obvious male cry as he pumps his semen into my husband's bottom.

Transgender

Jill, 29, Mother/Housewife

A recurring theme in my fantasies is wanking myself on to my partner's face, with his tongue flicking and slurping at the entrance to my hole. He loves to lap at my love juices and, I tell you, they really flow. Due to the early age at which I discovered my body, maybe five or six, I grew interested in new boys in town. At thirteen I saw my first porn movie. That was an amazing event. These days I still like passionate kisses; all hot and hurried. I love suggestive porn where you see a little and the rest is in your head. I love to hear moans and groans and my partner turns me on by letting me hear how much I've turned him on. Grabbing his cock really tight to stop him climaxing is brilliant. I love thinking about and seeing women making love together.

My favourite fantasy involves role-playing, as you will see. It is set in a nightclub with a gang of people. Suddenly the sexiest girl (Jed, my boyfriend, in some of my warm, worn, wet knickers, bra and dress or short skirt) comes over to where we are. She has to sit next to me (I am a man at this point). She is very quiet and shy; in fact a bit nervous. I start to talk to her, to make her feel at ease. I tell her how good she looks and how sexy she is. I feed her some line about coming back for coffee.

Once home I put on some slow music and we get closer and closer until finally we kiss, softly at first, round her neck and face, then more passionate. My hands start to slowly move over her shoulders and on to her tits. Then, very excitedly, I nose-dive, grabbing a tit and sucking and flicking her nipple. By this time she is starting to move and moan sexually. After a while I move my hand to her wanton pussy and stroke it softly and tenderly. (This is located underneath Jed's balls and before his hole.) I then proceed to slowly kiss and lick my way down her beautiful body, until I reach her clit. Then I lick and flick, like on a real clit. I flick my tongue about her hole and then suddenly ram it in. She squirms with delight at this. By this time we are both so hot and horny that I lob out my cock (an anal-penetration dildo, to be slotted on a penis for anal use) and start to wank my cock with Vaseline and baby oil mixed together. All the time I am licking her pussy and clit, then I slowly insert my cock into her tight wet hole and push in and out slowly, to let her get used to it.

Then I get a bit carried away and really fuck her hard and proper, banging against her. (Jed enjoys this game very much, so much by now that he's usually stopped and grabbed his own cock tightly to prevent ejaculation.) This is almost too much for her and we have to rest. When ready, we continue with me fucking her. We sometimes vary this fantasy and I'm a woman who introduces Jed to lesbian love.

Astrid, 29, Artist
Ever since *The Crying Game* my main fantasy has always been about making love to a hermaphrodite – and sometimes two hermaphrodites at once. I can think of nothing sexier than to be sucking on someone's tits, feeling the soft curves, and then reaching down and gripping a big, stiff cock.

In my favourite double-sexed fantasy I am in the middle of a park, sitting on the lush green grass in the middle of the day, while the sun beats down from above. There is no one else there and as I start to relax in the sunshine I take off all my clothes. I start to get really aroused and juicy lying there naked in the sunshine, but I feel very safe and relaxed.

Eventually I open my eyes. I can see a lady walking towards me; a beautiful woman wearing a gold and scarlet sari. I smile and at her and when she reaches me she sits down, too. She does not seem surprised that I am naked and after some small talk we start kissing. Our kisses soon become deep and wet and I lie on top of her. I run my hands over her breasts, which are big and full. I think I can feel something hard where her cunt is, but I know that's impossible. She takes off her beautiful sari, and I finally see the truth. S/he has two sets of genitals: a hard, dripping cock and a wet, sexy pussy as well. I go down on this beautiful person and lick and lick at his cunt, and when I'm tired I suck her cock. Whenever I get bored with one I switch and I feel as horny as when I started. Then she fucks me with her cock and at the same time I reach my hand down deep inside her pussy, so he gets fucked at the same time by me as well. I come and

110

so does my fantasy mate, creaming over from both cock and cunt.

When I dream about two hermaphrodites at once, it's usually the same scenario, except this time it's a man who approaches me across the green grass. He's got a beautiful pussy, which I discover when he asks me to go down on him, and then we are joined by the beautiful sari-woman and we all make wonderful love together; three hot pussies and two hard cocks.

Chapter Five
The Sexual Submissive

We now come to a category that is reflected in a lot of Black Lace stories and has formed a large proportion of the readers' sexual fantasies: the sexually submissive woman to a dominant other, who is usually, but not always, male. Anita Phillips says, in her book *A Defence of Masochism*, 'In submission one is done to rather than doing, and in sexual submission one is done to by somebody who is exciting and attractive.'[1] Political correctness dictates that we are not supposed to have these fantasies any more. However, they remain popular and ubiquitous in women's erotic stories. Dominant men have filled the pages of romantic and historical fiction – products bought and read almost exclusively by women – so it is no surprise that these characters have found their way into erotica. In our real lives we want men who treat us with respect and kindness. But in our imaginations, for reasons I shall attempt to analyse, we still like to cast rugged and handsome types who are able to physically conquer us.

In the five years that Black Lace books have been in

print, only a handful of stories have been submitted featuring sexually dominant female characters. This has surprised me. I thought that, given the opportunity, women would want to redress the balance and that an army of whip-wielding mistresses ready for battle would leap on to the pages, capture the male characters and subject them to all manner of ritual humiliations and exquisite tortures. Not so. While Black Lace heroines are assertive and independent, usually career women, they like their men to be potent, virile and sexually dominant. We printed questionnaires in the back of all Black Lace books, giving our readers a choice of qualities they preferred in their male characters: shy or sexually submissive men were actively disliked. It is interesting that the sexually dominant woman   the classic dominatrix figure – usually appears in female fantasy as a polysexual being whose purpose is to seduce the central female character or to act as a procuress for her. Changes in society and in the ways people think occur over long periods of time. It will take more than a few years of women's erotica being around before we exorcise Mr Darcy, Mr Rochester and all the other dark barons of women's literature. They seem to be our indulgence, in much the same way as the pneumatic multi-orgasmic blonde is for men. We feel comfortable with our clichés.

So where does the desire for sexual dominance come from? Most of us – men *and* women – are fearful of rejection and protective of our egos. Also, as we are all working so hard, it is quite nice to treat ourselves to the reverie of effortless pleasure. Anita Phillips comments: 'Sexual [submission] offers a way through for people who push themselves too hard, who over-achieve, who are never good enough; it gives an alternative to the impossible advice to take it easy.'[2] Or, in the words of Abbie's fantasy, 'As a lazy sort of person, it might just be a good way to receive lots of pleasure without too much work!' How wonderful to have a lover who knows what you want without you having to ask for it.

The Victorian sexologists made a pathology of sexual preference. They were keen to categorise different types of sexual behaviour in much the same way as explorers labelled new discoveries of insect or plant. To Krafft-Ebing and Freud, you were either normal or abnormal. And if you had a predilection for masochism or being dominated you were, most definitely, abnormal. Interestingly, their focus was on male submissives as the aberrant party; at the turn of the century female submission was taken as a given. And this is where I find a key to understanding submissive sexuality: if you are saddled with a lot of responsibility in your day-to-day life, it's a relief to leave your identity behind for a short while; to enjoy the escapism of letting someone else take control of your pleasure. The image of the successful businessman visiting a dominatrix is a cliché that has been used in a multitude of media. The reverse of this – the independent woman surrendering herself to the sexual lust of a physically imposing man – is an absolute taboo, however. We never think of the submissive male as being in danger, or that his sexuality is a false consciousness, but seeing a woman in this position makes us uncomfortable. This is partly because we are not used to thinking that men can be trusted with sexual power, and partly because we don't want to be seen reaffirming the old idea that women are naturally masochistic.

The biological determinism that evolved with Darwinist thinking claimed that men are the 'naturally dominant' gender. This opinion served as a blueprint for this century's social engineering and left little room for women to enjoy lives that freed them from childbearing and drudgery. Feminism has done much to liberate us from positions of social inferiority. And, as Anita Phillips points out, 'The notion of human beings as just another species with similar drives, impulses and sexual patterns to the animal kingdom . . . has only recently been challenged by post-war French thought. The latter emphasises the crucial nature of language to our culture – language which separates us from the animal kingdom.'[3]

With the advances in technology, education, automation and better communications, the traditional roles ascribed to gender are largely meaningless in the West. Women still bear children, but we are not dependent on men to hunt and kill our food and provide us with shelter and protection. The idea of the muscle-bound man throwing his weight around seems camp rather than threatening. The topical discussion as we approach the millennium is the function men serve these days, when strength isn't as crucial a requirement as mental dexterity and swift intellect. Girls are outshining boys in many subjects in the classroom, and the inequality that was accepted in our society as recently as forty years ago is becoming as quaint as the wind-up gramophone. We can even begin to play with the 'retro' qualities of outmoded rules. Look at the popularity of 'cheesecake' postcards and kitsch 40s and 50s 'girlie' images. The women in these products are fully made-up, buxom bombshells who exude sexiness and are usually featured in poses that exaggerate their form, thrust forward on high-heeled furry mules and scantily clad in diaphanous negligées. Interestingly, these images tend to be more popular with women than with today's heterosexual man. I suspect this is partly because the desirable body shape for 40s and 50s women was a fuller figure, and partly because we are visually literate enough to realise that we can have fun with the irony value of old stereotypes.

* * *

Many of the fantasies in the following section would be labelled by some people as rape fantasies, a term I believe is misleading. None of the fantasies that fit into this category are about being wounded, traumatised or half-killed. Similar to Nancy Friday's findings in *Women on Top*, I have never encountered a woman who said she really wanted to be raped. Friday's analysis of the term is that it was used as a way of getting around the guilt aspect of being a woman who craves sex. We would rather apportion blame to someone else than admit to desires we weren't supposed to have. While I believe this opinion is valid, I think the popularity of the submissive fantasy is more about preferring that someone else do all the hard work. Narcissism cannot be ruled out, either. All the women I spoke to agreed that the idea of a fantasy lover or favourite film star being unable to control his desire for you was a more realistic interpretation of the so-called rape fantasy. He is so hot for you – you are so desirable – that he is going to have to have you even if it means using force.

I try to get people to use the term submissive or narcissistic fantasy instead of the word rape. However, some women have said that the word itself can be arousing because it is so forbidden. While this will be offensive to anyone who has suffered because of rape, I don't think I have the right to tell a 42-year-old woman what she should and shouldn't be thinking about in the privacy of her own room.

The Dark Man of the Psyche

Submissive sexual fantasies are often very elaborate, requiring extensive mental set dressing. Looking at the deeper psychological reasons for our fascination with dark and disturbing elements in the stories we tell ourselves, it's useful to go back to childhood; to the first narratives we heard. Most of us are fortunate enough to grow up being allowed a rich fantasy life for the first few years of our lives. Before we have to knuckle down to the day-to-day routine of school, it's a non-stop world of narrative entertainment, most of it rooted in non-naturalistic realms. As children our imaginations become inhabited by a cast of archetypes, many of whose origins lie in the folklore of our ancestors and whose characteristics haven't changed that much through the centuries. There are more similarities than differences between *Beowulf* and *Power Rangers*. Many children's stories, films and cartoons combine elements of terror and beauty, chase and capture, imprisonment and escape, and are often imbued with a potency that stays in our minds' dressing-up box. Freud said, 'As people grow up, they cease to play, and they seem to give up the yield of pleasure which they gained from playing. But whoever understands the human mind knows that nothing is harder for a man than to give up a pleasure which he has once experienced.'[4]

Forgetting his sexism for a moment, the basic principle holds true. The stories that leave the biggest imprint on us – and the ones that are often the most enjoyable – are those that have the ability to scare us. As Michelle Olley has observed, 'Traditional fairy tales have always skated on the thin ice between the things we fear and the things we desire.'[5] Think of *Beauty and the Beast*, *Little Red Riding Hood*, *Snow White*, *Cinderella*, and the sexual sub-text of many of Grimm's fairy tales. Olley continues, 'Fairytale characters are early blueprints for SM icons.'[6] For instance, there is a large proportion of tyrants, overlords, dark masters, ice queens, princesses in peril, shape-shifters and superheroes in these stories. And the settings are often not that different from the backdrop to many classic stories of bondage and sadomasochism: palaces, castles, dungeons, forests. One example of this crossover is Anne

Rice's *Beauty* trilogy, erotic novels written under the pseudonym A N Roquelaure, where the famous author takes her virgin princess into a world of slavery and punishment, where misdemeanours are never overlooked and the exquisite reward of orgasm is always the flip side of erotic suffering.

No woman has explored the adult fairy tale more thoroughly and more eloquently than the late, great Angela Carter, whose fascination for Gothic tales, combined with her outstanding skill as a writer, produced works of lyrical exoticism. She said herself, 'I'd always been fond of ... Gothic tales, cruel tales, tales of wonder, tales of terror, fabulous narratives that deal directly with the imagery of the unconscious – mirrors; the externalised self; forsaken castles, haunted forests; forbidden sexual objects.'[7] Anyone who wants to investigate the female erotic imagination in literature would do well to read her work, particularly *The Bloody Chamber*, *Nights at the Circus*, *The Courtship of Mr Lyon* and *Wolf-Alice*. Mention must also be made of her non-fiction work, particularly *The Sadeian Woman*.

A similar process is at work in many of the fantasies in this book. Look at Tracey's story in the following section. She describes her first turn-ons as being movies about Romans, such as *Hercules*, or films where beautiful slave girls are captured and beaten. She goes on to stress that in real life she is the kindest person she knows, and she wouldn't want to hurt anyone. The archetypes in Tracey's fantasy are figures who could have been cast by Cecil B de Mille. We know that life in ancient times was nasty, brutish and short, but our imaginations conveniently dispel the ugly realities of poor hygiene and disease to go on to create an idealised past: a mythical Middle Ages where everyone has sparkling teeth; a pirate ship inhabited by handsome wild adventurers who aren't really going to harm us. We learn to suspend disbelief when we are very young and this useful ability stays with us for the rest of our lives. It's what enables us to gain pleasure from watching films, reading novels and going to the theatre. We need our collective dreaming. It's important to a sense of wellbeing and a key to finding out who we are. Without memory or imagination we are reduced as human beings.

Our sexual fantasies, too, are a form of collective dreaming. Again, there seem to be more similarities than differences. Although the characters we cast as the 'dominant other' may vary from person to person, we have a tendency to share cultural archetypes; for instance, the Mr Darcy figure from *Pride and Prejudice*. We like to think our fantasies are unique and we often feel ashamed of them; we want them to remain secret. Freud said that man cherishes his fantasies as his most intimate possessions and is more comfortable to confess his misdeeds than his innermost thoughts. He went on, however, to say that only an unsatisfied person fantasises and that to confess to having daydreams – erotic or otherwise – was tantamount to admitting to one's inadequacies. It is ironic that the period in which Freud was working saw the beginning of the greatest explosion of products of the fantastic imagination through the invention of the cinema, not to mention the stories of Lewis Carroll.

Luckily, we are not so guilt-ridden today that we have to wave goodbye to the secret realm of our fantasies as we grow up. Confessing to having daydreams is proof that you have an active, creative imagination, and it is not so unusual if some of your thoughts are dark and flirt with taboos. Our subconscious will throw up all manner of scary monsters as a means of getting us used to dealing with danger. We can gain a lot of pleasure and knowledge about ourselves by working through our fantasies and not being ashamed of them. Tackling our demons by sexualising them is healthier than sweeping them under the carpet. 'To understand the predator' – what Clarissa Pinkola Estés calls the 'dark man' – 'of our psyche is to become a mature animal who is not vulnerable out of naivete, inexperience, or foolishness.'[8]

If we are controlling the dark man, then he isn't a threat to us; he serves as an instrument for our pleasure. We can choose when to bring him into our fantasies, and we can banish him when he is no longer a potent archetype. Sexual fantasies need not be static. What excites us now may lose its fascination in ten or twenty years' time. As we grow older and move further away from the fairy-tale world of demons and princesses, different characters may appear in our sexual imaginations. Sexual archetypes can tell us about who we are and where we are in our lives. This is why it's important to discuss the taboo fantasies of sexual submission. Far from being a false consciousness, they are a way for women to unlock the mysteries of the wild unconscious. Have no guilt – unless it turns you on!

Lesley, 32, Manager

My fantasies run along the lines of being dominated, forced and abused – never nastily, but forcefully. I fantasise about tall, strong, quiet and mysterious men: strangers, or Rutger Hauer or Marti Pellow. I had a very repressed sexual childhood and was told that good girls just didn't 'do it'. As soon as I was an adult I tried all sorts. I'm quite independent, somewhat cuddly in shape, and like a strong man – not a wimp! I always have to take the lead in everyday life, so I look for the opposite in sex.

I think about meeting a tall, strong male at a disco or pub or conference. After being taken for a drink and being chatted up, I am taken back to his place and forcibly kissed and groped. I am reluctant but at the same time excited. He suggests going further and I agree. He leads me to the bedroom. There are restraints lying on the bed. He explains that before sex he needs to inspect me to ensure I'm OK. He chains me to the bed, knees up and legs apart, and starts inspecting, fondling, probing, licking. Compliments abound. He issues me with instructions such as 'Open wider'. After my inspection he says, 'Wonderful. Now let's see what you're really made of.' Then, basically, anything goes: me giving blow jobs as he rams fingers and a dildo in my pussy and beads in my anus, and then a larger dildo in my pussy. He also uses nipple clamps. I am made to use various phallic objects. Finally I'm taken from behind – roughly. I wish I could stay with him for weeks! After all that we kiss and cuddle and drink some wine and have polite conversation. He suggests we meet again; he has a friend he would like to introduce me to.

Maxine, 19, Student
When I was little I used to fancy Luke Skywalker from *Star Wars*. Now I think of naughty things like threesomes or being groped or shagging in public. One-night stands used to be my bag; the detachedness of them is great. My recurring fantasies are of being powerless or being had by more than one man at once.

My favourite fantasy is that after a raging argument, my lover hides in my flat. I come home from a party dressed very skimpily and in the darkness he grabs me from behind, puts his arm around my neck and warns me not to scream. He then throws me over the back of the sofa and severely fucks me from behind, teasing me by letting his huge cock slither up my arse. I'm left sore and throbbing and tingling all over. Then he carries me to the bed, kisses me gently and makes love to me slowly. He comes inside me and then we fall asleep in each other's arms.

Rhianna, 28, Carer
My main thing is domination. I love being dominated in bed by strong husky men. Black guys are a big turn-on for me. I didn't really discover my sexuality until last year. When I was younger I had sex with a lot of guys, but that's all it was: sex. Last year I met somebody who showed me that sex wasn't the crux of a relationship; your minds and souls also had to mate.

I have always fantasised that I would be walking somewhere and I would meet a tall, dark handsome guy who would totally dominate me. He would take me back to his place and order me to take off my clothes. He would make me lean back against the wall and start to tease me with butterfly kisses, making me beg for his mouth and tongue. Once I had begged enough, he would give it to me, kissing me roughly, bruising my lips and exploring my mouth with his tongue. While he was kissing me his hands would be on my breasts, squeezing and tugging the nipples, making me feel pleasure/pain.

At this point I wanted him between my legs, his mouth sucking and nibbling at my clit, fucking me with his fingers. When I was at the point of orgasm, he would stop and sit down on the couch. He would sit me down in front of him and start playing with his cock. I would beg to touch it, stroke and suck it, and to play with his balls. Again, once I had begged enough he would let me suck him, nibble the head and try to swallow his cock. I tell him I want him to come in my mouth. At that point he slaps me. He lays me face down on the floor with a couple of pillows under my hips. He then lies down on top of me, teasing my cunt with his cock. Finally he plunges into me. I cry out in pleasure. He forces deep inside me, again and again until I can't bear it any more. He then rubs my clitoris, bringing me to orgasm. He keeps stoking his cock in me until he also orgasms. We both fall asleep this time, only to wake up and start all over again.

Abbie, 48, Computer Operator
I never had sex before I was married but I got a great deal of experience and pleasure out of wanking men off. Even now I'm totally addicted to playing with my husband's cock. I like oral sex, mutual masturbation, getting dressed up and, of course, reading Black Lace books; sometimes to get in the mood, or other times while my husband plays with me. He usually gives me an orgasm before we have intercourse.

My favourite fantasy is of being dominated. I imagine a historical setting. A girl is all alone and goes to a place such as a monastery, where she is offered shelter as long as she sells herself to them. She then has to learn obedience and discipline. At all times she is clothed in harnesses that are covered by long robes. Normally she is also wearing chains. At any time she can be made to strip and perform any act of sex on demand from her masters and mistresses. At all times, though, she gets as much satisfaction from it as they do. I think that by having a fantasy where somebody else has total control it takes away any guilt feelings and allows you to just enjoy what is going on. Mind you, as a lazy sort of person, it might just be a good way to receive lots of pleasure without too much work!

Joyce, 40, Admin Manager
I remember having strange dreams with masochistic tones when I was as young as four years old. I don't have one particular fantasy but they all centre around a naive, innocent or ordinary woman being forced into sexual slavery, as in *The Story of O*. My fantasies are all masochistic and sometimes involve anal sex and even animals.

Natalie, 26, Mother

My fantasy is that I am lost in a wood and dressed only in rags. I'm found by a woman and a man and taken back to a house where the woman takes me to wash and dress. However, she fastens me to a bed with handcuffs and begins to whip and dominate me. Her man-friend comes in and I am their sex slave, which involves dildos, oral and anal sex, food and nipple clamps.

Pat, 42, Retail Worker

My first turn-ons were books: *The Story of O* and any books including spanking, bondage and whips. For my fantasy I imagine we have met another couple at a prearranged pub where we swap partners for a weekend. I drive off with my partner and he stops in a secluded spot and screws me over the car. When he finds I'm wearing knickers he spanks me and, after ejaculating, he ties me up in the back of the car while his sperm is dripping down my legs. He then drives to this remote lodge and makes me perform oral sex on him, still tied up. After this he unties me and tells me to clean myself up and make sure I'm clean everywhere because he's going to fuck my arse next. This he proceeds to do for the entire weekend. I'm kept tied up and have to perform various dirty acts.

Rebecca, 44, Mature Student

I think *The Story of O* is the most erotic piece of writing ever. And when I discovered Henry Miller I realised that sexy writing was hidden away in books. This was what turned me on most – much more than TV or films.

I have a very submissive sexuality. Please note that this submissiveness is not apparent in any other area of my life. I am a strong-willed woman from a family of strong-willed women. I am intelligent and have worked in responsible positions in industry for 25 years.

I am totally monogamous and my husband is always the master in my fantasies. The keys to the eroticism in my fantasies are total submission, total obedience and total humility. This includes displaying myself in a sexual manner, discipline of various kinds and being treated as a sexual toy. Naturally, these fantasies go beyond anything that my husband and I actually do, but we enjoy acting out watered-down versions of them. By this I mean that they are symbolic, rather than being the cruelly described beatings in my fantasies, and we never do anything dangerous or harmful.

Tracey, 46, Health Worker
When I was young, my first turn-ons were movies about Romans, such as *Hercules*, or where a beautiful slave girl was captured and chained to the bars of a cage, stripped and beaten in front of her lover. The same kinds of things are turn-ons now and I also enjoy sex one hundred per cent more while or after looking at any kind of porn. Pictures are a favourite with me although I do dislike lesbian scenarios. However, I think my fantasies are maybe too sadistic to really go into detail. They always feature a submissive female. A victimised male is allowed as long as the 'cruel' party is male and a submissive or forced female is present to share the pain, which, of course, is the source of the pleasure. In real life I'm the kindest person I know. And I don't want to hurt anyone or be brutalised.

I am fascinated with male ejaculation and orgasms. I sometimes fantasise about brother–sister or father–daughter incest. However, this is a classic example where the realisation of the fantasy would not work. In fact, I hate the thought. In this fantasy, the 'brother' or 'father' is no more real than a vibrator is a 'man'.

Georgina, 37, Laundry Assistant

I can't think of anything specific which influenced me when I was younger but these days I like erotic fiction and certain music. 'Do I Have To Say The Words' by Bryan Adams makes me go weak at the knees. My fantasies usually involve several men making love to one woman – not always me – and the men vary. The only thing they have in common is that their erections last for ever!

One particular fantasy starts with a woman going into a lift. She is small and petite and is wearing a smart linen suit with a shortish skirt. When the lift stops at the next floor a huge black man gets in. He is six feet tall with broad shoulders and is very muscular. He has a key to override the lift controls and he uses it to stop the lift between floors. She asks him what the hell he is doing and he says that he wants to get himself a piece of white ass. She backs away as far as she can but he pins her up against the side of the lift. She struggles and scratches him but he just laughs and lifts her skirt up, rips her knickers away and proceeds to frig her relentlessly with his strong fingers. Her juices start to flow and he calls her names – whore, slut, etc., – and then, releasing his huge erection, proceeds to fuck her using all his strength to plough inside her.

This is usually as much as I need but, if I have to go on, after he has finished with her he restarts the lift and takes her back to his apartment where his three roommates take turns with her. This is just one of my fantasies. I find they get stale quickly and I know I'd hate anything like this to happen in real life. My current boyfriend doesn't feel threatened by my fantasies. In fact he encourages them on the grounds that anything that makes it good for me is good for him, too. This is unlike my ex, who found them insulting!

Abigail, 26, Hairdresser

Historical adventure books were always a big turn-on for me. They still are. Faceless men or men wearing crash helmets or tight masks also always do the trick. I find reading erotic fiction a big turn-on. I get turned on thinking about group sex; for example, me and three men. I like my fantasies to be set in the past.

My favourite fantasy is of being abducted by pirates and having my clothes cut off me with a sword. I'm then stripped or chained to a bed, kept naked and blindfolded until my favourite pirate decides to take me. I like to feel submissive but eager for any plans he may have for me. I also like imagining I'm a sex slave to my boyfriend, where he forces me to do things that I subconsciously want but could never ask for, such as having an audience while having sex or trying S&M.

Leila, 24, Occupation Unknown

Submission dominates my most recurring fantasies. I do not fantasise about plain old romantic sex nearly as often. I'm not sure my mind sees such a difference; in both sets of fantasies I see a strong male character, but there are two flavours. I am a big book reader, and I think I have an incredible imagination. When I started to be conscious of my sexual desires I started reading Jon Gorman's *GOR* novels, and *The Clan of the Cave Bear*. These days I like men who reek of testosterone and are broad shouldered. I like being reminded by looks, smiles and flirtations that I'm female. I think about being caught doing something naughty.

The fantasy I would like to share with you – my favourite – is that I have arrived in China to teach English. However, when I arrive there, I am kidnapped. I wake up in a room with no windows. I have no luggage, no wallet, no passport.

I wonder where I am. I can only speak conversational Chinese and won't be able to make anyone understand what's happened to me. I try the door but, of course, it's locked. I start to get a really bad feeling. I pound on the door but no one answers. Sometime later the door opens to admit four men. All of them are Asian; the first two are about my height and very muscular and sparsely dressed. The third is shorter and wearing very rich garments made from silk. The last one is taller and has on a very nice suit. The last two are speaking Chinese to each other.

'Where am I and what am I doing here?' I demand. They reply that it is of no consequence as it appears I will not be staying very long. Then the shorter man orders me to take off my clothes. I refuse, and twice he repeats his demand. He then brings out my passport and visa, holding a lighter in his other hand.

'What do you want from me?' I ask.

'I want you to take off your clothes.'

I look at the two burly men. They would have no problem in subduing me. So I start to take off my clothes. I feel very self-conscious, but I don't bother trying to cover myself up. The tall man calls me over. I had almost forgotten about him. He has been sitting leisurely, watching me.

'Put your feet either side of mine,' he commands in English, and he sits up and puts his feet in front of the legs of the chair. 'Bend your knees and put your hands behind your neck.'

This is my first real taste of fear. I hesitate and he reaches forward and hits the back of my thigh with the palm of his hand. I jump and do what he tells me. I am very conscious of how open and exposed I feel. He lets me feel that for a few moments, then his hand rests on my knee and he begins to move it up to my breast, where he runs his palm over my nipple and his fingertips over my collarbone. My nipple hardens and he

128

runs his hand over it a little more, making the other one ache for attention. His hand goes down across my stomach and starts to glide between my legs. I want to move but I can't.

'Look at me,' he says.

I open my eyes and look into his face. I feel so trapped. His hand slides between my legs and I know that he can feel the wet, slick feeling down there, which is getting wetter by the moment. He smiles a small smile. He starts to lubricate my clit with his juices and slowly rubs me there. I draw in a shuddering breath and try to control the urge to move my hips. All I can think about is, I don't want the others to know I am enjoying this and how much I want him to continue.

'Please stop,' I ask.

He smacks my thigh again, and this time I lose balance and steady myself by putting my hands on his shoulders. He stops moving his fingers but leaves them between my legs. I cannot control the urge to move my hips. With his free hand, he grabs my long hair and pulls my head down to his.

'I know you don't really want me to stop, but I will, because you don't want me to,' he whispers in my ear. Shivers run down my spine.

'Thank you,' I say.

'Thank you, sir,' he corrects.

His hand caresses me one more time before he tells me to go and sit down. I want to curl up on the bed, but I am sure I won't be allowed to. I'm aware of the rumours of white slavery but I hadn't thought I would be in danger. The tall man starts speaking to the shorter one and discussing money. He says, '*Duoshao qian*?' which means, 'How much?'

This is only the beginning of several fantasies in which I am a slave in a remote part of China, and I can't leave because I have no money and no passport.

Deborah, 32, Nursery Nurse

I always liked the idea of discovery; having sex with the possibility of being caught. I like to imagine a slave at a posh dinner party. She is the mistress of the baron and is ordered to undress before his elderly guests and is then blindfolded and spread-eagled on a bed and serviced by a large black man, a young woman and then by the guests, starting with an elderly woman. The baron sits in an armchair and watches. There are no holds barred. The guests can do to her whatever they wish, and she cannot refuse and must do what they want.

Laura, 31, Guest House Owner

When I was about fifteen, I used to imagine I had been kidnapped by a tall dark gypsy with one of those nicely painted wooden horse-drawn caravans. He would keep me locked inside, travelling all day and being a sex slave by night. I don't know how this fantasy ended as I never imagined an ending. I met my husband at sixteen and the fantasies stopped.

Sylvia, 21, Student

When I was much younger I found a copy of a kinky US magazine in an abandoned house. It covered themes such as group sex, anal sex and S&M. I had by this time already achieved orgasm with my electric toothbrush. The discovery of the magazine expanded my sexual fantasy range from common sex to the more kinky side, including bondage, spanking and an extreme fetish with anal sex. I read the *Hite Report* the next year and would masturbate to the sections on anal sex. Leather and vinyl clothing titillated my young mind, as well as the sex columns in women's magazines. As I became more sexually experienced, my fascination with extremes faded. Women's bodies are one of the biggest turn-ons for me, but not displayed in an explicit or pornographic way. Large men are a weakness of mine, as well as satin, silk or anything that feels sensual on the skin.

Being the self-confident, successful person I am, many of my fantasies revolve around being dominated. In my fantasies, I don't become submissive as such, but am confronted with real strength (something not always found in men with excessive physical strength), sexual confidence and seductive techniques. Someone who makes me feel like a woman without losing my power. My current fantasy revolves around being kidnapped by my lover and taken to a beautiful place I have never been to and being forced to fulfil his/her dirtiest sexual desires.

Denise, 36, Health Shop Manager

My recurring fantasies involve being bound or shaved and having no power and being on show to many. Different things at different times can turn me on, depending on my mood, but my earliest turn-on was watching a man slowly remove his shirt. My favourite fantasy now is that I arrange to meet a friend but, during the journey, I'm kidnapped by a group of people. Some of them are masked but all are strangers. I'm then taken to an isolated country house, where I am pushed into the hall and surrounded by many people. A voice orders me to strip. I refuse, but I am undressed. Once naked I am paraded for all to see towards a platform. They lay me down and I am shaved all over and am totally hairless. Then many hands are all over me. I am moved into various positions so people can gain access to all places. Sexual toys are placed inside me, then men replace the toys, until everyone climaxes. I am kept prisoner for what seems like many days but when I'm released I find out that only a few hours have passed.

Sally, 29, Mother
I've always found historical romance a turn-on, and romantic sex scenes in films such as *An Officer and a Gentlemen* or *The Big Easy*. Now, sex needs to have more graphic words and pictures. I have a few hard-core porn films, which are good, and I like using a vibrator. Anal sex is a turn-on because it is slightly uncomfortable. The recurring themes in my fantasies are of sexual activity with and corporal punishment of teenagers, or being kept as a sex prisoner or slave. My fantasies tend to have historical or Far East settings; for example, set in the Victorian period or in a harem. I find the whole idea of being cleaned internally followed by anal sex arousing. I like the idea of being beaten into sexual submission – but only in my imagination! I've tried to write down my fantasy, but I find to go into too much detail makes it too real and it loses its effect. The unreality is what's important to me.

Nina, 40, Housewife
I think about bondage, humiliation and domination. I fantasise that I'm in prison – why, I don't know – and that I'm being stripped and searched by the wardens and the governor. I have to be examined inside and out, then put into a room with other women who are testing out various sexual aids/equipment as part of their punishment.

Jenni, 24, Mother
When I was younger I used to find people who worked on fairgrounds a turn-on; people with greasy grubby clothes who were really rough. These days it's anyone I can't have, and people who are very domineering and not afraid to try something new and who take the lead.

My fantasy is that I'm sitting with two male friends having dinner when they put sleeping tablets in my food without me knowing. They then wait until I pass out, and take it in turns to have sex with me. Then they do it together, then by using vegetables and vibrators to make me come. They clean and dress me and, when I come back round, they ask me if I'm all right. They tell me I fainted and I'm none the wiser.

Lenore, 30, Unemployed

I always went for what I thought was normal. I never experimented with sex until I got older. When I saw films about a woman having sex with two men, it really aroused me; so did the idea of being tied up while men had sex with me. I like the idea of a dominant male, someone who will take control of the situation. My fantasies are most often about me having sex with two men or being punished, abused or tied up, or being put into prostitution or bondage.

My favourite fantasy is that I don't know where I am. I end up being in a room on a sacrificial table. I feel drowsy. I see men; they are all naked. There's a guy at the end of the table, who says that I am to be an object of pleasure to all the men. But first, he's going to start the ceremony by fucking me. He takes his dick in his hand and spreads my legs, then pushes me forward and enters me. I feel pain, but pleasure. He tells me that the men are going to use me in any way they want. I'm going to be fucked and abused until I'm sore. I'm going to be abused with vibrators, dildos and toys. I'm going to be tied up and fucked back and front by two men. I'm going to be raped and taken when I least expect it.

After he has fucked me, he tells his congregation to come and drink the juices of the sacrifice. So they all file up to lick my fanny one by one. After this I'm transported into a room with gadgets and a bed. This is the room where I am to be continually fucked until I'm exhausted and unable to move.

Diana, 42, Housewife

I have always been out with older men. When I was younger I read a great deal of *True Confessions* magazines. I used to strip in front of my bedroom window, knowing the man across the street was watching. At that age the danger of being caught was exciting. These days I enjoy reading about forbidden relationships such as nuns with priests, or incest. I like training books for BDSM and the smell of aftershave, the ocean and rain.

Male dominance is the primary factor in my fantasies, and even rape, or being held captive in the Far East in a harem. I always think about an older, strong, handsome man. He has a tender heart, but he knows instinctively when no doesn't mean no. Sometimes he brings a partner in; for example, a masseuse – sometimes a man, sometimes a woman. They would massage normally at first but then it gets erotic and the man would watch as the masseuse masturbates me to orgasm. They are then both so aroused that they fuck like crazy.

I think about a doctor's examination that is very thorough and includes medical procedures such as an enema. Or that I'm being pulled over in a strange town and I get arrested for nothing. The cop forces me to go through a strip search. Anal sex is intriguing. It seems that dominance over me is the main theme.

Trudy, 26, Admin Assistant

I was eleven when I first noticed my body changing. I really liked the actor Patrick Duffy, the star of *Dallas*, and I would lie awake at night thinking about him, wondering what it would be like to lie in his arms. I would imagine that we would get married. I still like hairy chests and nice eyes! These days, it's David Duchovny, or someone with an incredible voice and strong hands. Having a back massage and long, slow kisses turn me on. The recurring theme in my fantasies, however, is that there is more than one man and I am being watched as I perform any number of sexual acts. Sometimes I am being held down and forced to endure what is little more than rape. But it doesn't feel degrading and there is no real fear involved. I have control during the fantasy.

Here is my favourite fantasy. It is late at night and I am tired. I am offered a lift that I know is dangerous to accept but I accept it anyway. The face of the driver changes depending on who I fancy that week. I feel unthreatened and unafraid. We talk about a lot of things. At this point the fantasy goes one of two ways. If I've had a good day I'm the one to initiate sex. In the other version, he takes me to a motel or his house and forces me into his bedroom. I am stripped and he uses gutter language to tell me in detail what he wants to do and how he's going to take me.

Admitting that I want it is never a part of the fantasy, even when he's supposed to make me beg. If I'm having a really bad day, it's the man who is forced into sex by me, as if I can control my own life through my fantasy one. None of it is real rape, though. I am never injured in my fantasies; in no way am I hurt. Sometimes a friend re-enacts my fantasy for me, but that's a different story!

Chapter Six

Bondage, Punishment and all the Trimmings

Thou hast not half the power to do me harm
As I have to be hurt.
William Shakespeare, *Othello* (1602–4)

*M*uch of the analysis pertinent to this section is covered in the introduction to the section on submissive sexuality. What is different about the fantasies in this category is the elaborate set dressing and the paraphernalia of punishment. All the whips, straps, racks, belts and handcuffs lend a theatricality to the scenario. Similar to the medical fantasies, the details are important here, and the sophistication of the imagination is immediately apparent. The first fantasy has its subject held in fur-lined leather wrist and ankle restraints while she admires the fresco on the ceiling before listening to Chopin's *Nocturne* in the half-light of a Gothic chamber. Later in the section, the spanking fantasies are less elaborate in their set dressing, but the anticipation of waiting for the punishment is as torturous and exquisite as that in the most elaborate of scenarios.

Many feminists feel apprehensive (and downright appalled) by the fact that some women enjoy SM fantasy from the submissive position. Their argument says that by gaining pleasure from a traditional position of inequality means that we are labouring under a false consciousness: Avis Lewallen describes us as being 'Caught up within patriarchal systems, and actively desiring within them.'[1] However, playing a part in the bedroom doesn't mean we are surrendering our rights in society. We are not choosing to give up our rights as employees, citizens or individuals. This is exemplified by the fact that many lesbian couples are active in the SM scene. Who is the one in denial when a pro-censorship feminist tells a happily out and proud daddy dyke that her sexuality is a false consciousness? The simple fact is that some people like to perform; to act out a private theatre with their partner. As educated grown-ups I think we can decide for ourselves which games we like to play in the privacy of our own homes. We can have fun with stereotypes, and dressing up is an important part of this theatre. It could be said that having fun with stereotypes is an insult in a world where inequality is rife. By this token it is also unfair to take public holidays, eat healthily and have access to sanitation and modern medicine. The sexual arena is not where these inequalities should be tackled. Imbalances of power occur where there are imbalances of wealth, and this book is about the politics of pleasure, not economics.

Most sadomasochistic relationships are consensual and based on trust; nearly all couples into SM have a safe word that remains sacred. When the word is uttered, the play stops. I want to make one thing clear: having consensual sex where one person plays the dominant party has nothing to do with domestic violence, which is a crime. SM-ers are responsible people, and there are many UK and US organisations that provide support and safety guidelines to people interested in experimenting with this side of their sexuality. It would be foolish to leap straight into SM sex without knowing the person and talking over beforehand what you are both into. Any responsible person in the SM scene would recommend that a novice equip her/himself in the basics of how to tie up your partner safely (if you're into bondage), or how the various instruments of correction deliver different results (if you're into punishment). Addresses are given in the back of this book where you can find out more information.

Many submissives in the scene write down their sexual wishes, and the dominant partner goes to great lengths to create an environment that will fulfil their partner's wildest dreams. Getting all the clothes, props and environment sorted out is something of a labour of love, and the dominant half of a sub-dom partnership is by far the hardest work. One way of looking at SM practice is that it is cowboys and Indians for adults. The excitement of chase, capture, imprisonment and confession is something we learn from our childhood games. Having a loving partner tie us up and punish us is not too great a leap from the playground games of our childhood. Remember the girls screaming with excitement when a game of kisschase was on the cards? Some of us don't grow out of wanting these games; we just swap the playground for the bedroom.

There is a huge difference between being a victim and being a willing submissive. A victim is someone who has no choice over what is happening to her/him. A real-life masochist or willing submissive has initiated a complex power exchange between her/himself and a consenting partner. A fantasy dominant is an archetype the fantasist has cast in her own narrative. The victim status connotes pleasure, and the events – however extreme – that transpire in that fantasy are controlled by her.

Anon, 38, Doctor
I like the erotic possibilities that a dental chair conjures in my mind. I also find arousing the idea of being gently stretched on a rack and pleasured. Imagining the pleasure a vibrator can give is a turn-on, too. I also used to get off on wearing hot pants with crossover straps but now I prefer silk pyjamas. Bondage scenes and, to the other extreme, long, slow massages are sexy.

My favourite fantasy begins while I am asleep in the guest room of a private castle. I hear the door opening, and a woman dressed in a simple grey belted uniform of a servant enters. She is followed by two manservants dressed in black. She quietly but firmly orders me out of bed and to follow her. I do not question her. The two male attendants follow not far behind. I am wearing my ivory silk and satin shorts and a short-sleeved pyjama jacket. I am led into a dimly lit room in the castle basement. There is a low vaulted ceiling with a fresco, but the light is too dim to make out the details.

Firm hands on either side lead me towards the middle of the room, where two chains hang down from bolts set in the ceiling. On the end of each chain is a soft leather cuff. The two male attendants continue to hold each of my shoulders, and the female attendant walks in front of me. She has a large bunch of keys attached to a ring on her belt, and it jangles slightly as she moves. She begins to undo the buttons of my pyjama jacket, starting at the top, working down slowly and deliberately pausing between each button. The male attendants pull the jacket back over my shoulders and pass it to the female attendant, who places it on some kind of table at the far end of the room in front of me.

'Put her arms up,' she orders. The male attendants fasten my wrists into place. The female walks towards me and looks at my satin shorts. To my relief, she doesn't remove them but starts to push my feet apart. The two male attendants kneel down, each grasping one ankle, which they pull outward and attach via leather cuffs to metal rings set into the smooth stone-flagged floor. No words are uttered, and all three walk behind me. I hear them leaving the chamber, closing the door with a loud bang. The key is turned in the lock and I am all alone.

The wrist restraints are firm, but there is enough give for me to pull my arms out if I really want to. I remain in place and my eyes become gradually accustomed to the dark. Above on the ceiling are cherubs at play, gambolling on soft, fluffy clouds, while others play musical instruments. At the far end of the room, a lone cherub sits cross-legged, playing with his distinctly non-cherubic phallus. He seems to be directing a knowing look towards me. To my left there is a metal grill leading to a small chamber. Behind the metal bars, I can make out an antique dental chair, lit by a soft overhead spotlight. I can just see that it is upholstered in purple crushed velvet. It has black leather straps attached to each armrest. The footrest is in two widely separated halves, with further straps to hold the victim in delicious anticipation. On the table by the chair are various instruments, which are definitely not dental.

To my right is another metal grill door, leading to another, larger antechamber. My eyes focus on a functional medieval rack, with rollers and ankle restraints connected to a spreader bar at the end nearest to me. The table seems to be softly upholstered in black leather, and the straps attached to the rollers are made of plaited pink leather. At the far end of the main

140

chamber is a small table with simple wooden chairs. There is a narrow archway in the wall behind the desk, leading up some stone steps that disappear into the darkness towards the master's quarters. I know that whatever fate awaits me lies at the top of the stairs.

I wait for some time in the semi-darkness, then hear the sound of a piano coming from upstairs: Chopin's *Nocturne*, my favourite. The playing is immaculate and goes on for twenty minutes or so before the piano lid is slammed shut. I hear the sound of footsteps slowly descending the stairs. I tug on the restraints, but not hard enough to escape. Butterflies flutter in my stomach. Finally a tall figure steps into the room. He is dressed in knee-length leather boots, tight britches and a white shirt with ties at the front. He has black unruly hair and piercing blue eyes. He steps towards me and I notice he has a riding crop in his right hand. He strokes the tip of it along my crotch, just pushing the material into my moist cleft; then he lifts my left breast with the tip.

'I hope you like my room. My ancestors had vivid imaginations and I've added a few touches of my own,' he says, glancing towards the dental chair. 'Don't worry, they were harmless, mostly, and so am I – mostly.' He then walks round behind me and presses his body into mine. I can feel his large erection pressing into my back, as his hands move round to cup my breasts. He pinches my nipples between thumb and forefingers, planting soft kisses on my neck. Next, his hands move slowly down, pushing under the elasticated waist of my shorts. I can feel his fingers creeping through my pubic curls, seeking out what he is looking for. I feel him spreading my labia, brushing against my clitoris, then he enters my cunt with a single finger. It is promptly withdrawn and held to his nose.

'I see I'm not holding you entirely against your will,' he says with a smile. I don't reply. He then goes to the table and pours himself a large brandy from a dust-covered bottle. He watches me as he slowly drinks. I pull on the restraints. 'Oh, don't pull too hard, you might free yourself. You wouldn't want that, would you?'

'No,' I admit softly.

He continues to stare at me and, above him, the obscene cherub seems to leer at me, increasing my discomfort. After a time he puts down his brandy and walks towards the metal grill to my left. He moves as if to open the door leading to the dental chair, but changes his mind. He walks, instead, to another door leading to a rack. He walks in and lights candles set into recesses in the room, filling the chamber with a warm flickering light. He comes towards me, kneels on the floor and undoes the ankle restraints. He pauses and pushes the material of my satin shorts into my crotch and plants a lingering kiss through the material. Then he starts to pull the shorts down to the floor. I pull each leg out in turn; he picks up the shorts and examines and sniffs the damp patch in the material. I long for him to apply his mouth to my private parts but, instead, he reaches up and undoes the wrist restraints and leads me through the open door towards the rack.

No words are exchanged. He gently thwacks the upholstered surface of the rack with his riding crop and indicates with the briefest, slightest turn of his head that I am to climb on to the padded surface. I comply, offering no protest or resistance. I sit on the rack, supported by my hands stretched out behind me, with my knees slightly bent. He takes one ankle at a time and secures it to one end of the spreader bar with broad, soft leather straps. I am now sitting semi-upright with my legs stretched wide apart. It is not a comfortable position but I cannot take my eyes from him. He attaches the rope in the middle of the spreader bar to a cleat in the far end of the table.

Then he gently pushes me back against the table so that I am flat on my back, looking at the ceiling. He attaches my wrists to the leather straps, so that my arms are pulled above my head. I imagine serving wenches brought down to the chamber in ages past, offering only half-hearted resistance and being stripped and secured to the same instrument of pain and pleasure. My thoughts soon return to the here and now, as he pulls the lever operating the rollers to which my wrists are attached. I hear the ratchet engaging and the creaking sounds of the plaited leather straps tightening against each other. My arms are pulled straight, and my body slides up the table slightly. He continues to pull, and my body feels taut and my skin deliciously stretched. I begin to wonder whether the stretching will continue to the point of pain, when the safety mechanism cuts in and the rack stops tightening.

'Mmm,' he mutters. 'An ingenious mechanism to stop me getting carried away – pity.' I am stretched out so that I can only move my head from side to side and wiggle my fingers and toes. I look up at the ceiling, where countless previous captives must have stared with fear and anticipation. A faint outline of the same leering cherub is visible. I feel a sense of communion with the past captives.

My master takes a small white feather and traces delicate circles on the inside of my wrist, inside my arm, and over my shoulder towards my breasts. Then he – oh so delicately – circles my areolae with the lightest touch of the feather, before proceeding down my abdomen towards my pubis. He skirts around my curls to the kissable skin on the inside of my thighs and down towards my ankles. My skin feels tight and super-sensitive to even the slightest touch. He drops the feather and begins to gently massage my breasts slowly, increasing in tempo and vigour, finally giving my nipples a firm and slightly painful squeeze.

Next, he moves to one of the alcoves and removes a candle, which he holds above my breasts. The flickering light of the candle casts demonic shadows of my tormentor on to the wall. He waits and waits, and I see molten wax building up in the hollow around the wick. It can only be a moment until it runs down the side of the candle on to my breasts. Then he slowly and deliberately tilts the candle, directing a stream of hot wax on to one nipple. I gasp with pleasure and pain, pushing my head back into the upholstered surface of the rack. He looks down on me with a soft mocking smile, pauses, waiting for more wax to collect, and repeats the process on the other side. He picks off the solidified wax with his fingernails, gently scratching my erect nipples in the process. He repeats the process several times until the effect starts to wear off.

Next, he moves another lever, which causes a leather pad to push upwards against my bottom, pushing my pubic bone up, exposing and opening me up to his intense gaze. He kisses the inside of my thighs. I can feel his hot breath on my clitoris, then I feel him spreading my labia with his fingers and stroking his tongue along the engorged flesh over and over again. He finally gets to my clitoris, licks it, and I am nearly lost. I long for him to continue but, instead, he enters me with his finger and spreads my secretions along my labia. He stops to take something from a small recess in the wall. It is a large, smooth, stone phallus.

'We found this when we excavated the moat,' he says with a smile. He starts to spread my secretions on to the bulbous head, then gently slides the tip along my labia before pushing the bulbous head inside me. He pauses, then slowly inserts the phallus deeper and deeper until I am completely filled and stretched. He works the phallus until its base just touches my clitoris each time. Finally, when I am close to the brink, he withdraws the phallus and stops. I expect him to move on to some other torment but, instead, he undoes the straps around my ankles and my wrists. He gently lifts my stretched and tender body off the rack and cradles me in his strong arms. He carries me out of the chamber and up the stairs to his bedroom in the castle keep, where we are to spend the night and where I will finally find release.

Simona, 18, Student
I have always been turned on by fantasies of sex with women, particularly good-looking ones who wouldn't want to have sex with me. Bondage and slave scenes are also my favourites. These types of fantasies go back a long way, perhaps to when I was ten years old. A particular favourite scenario goes like this: I am handcuffed to the bed and have to give in to anything my partner wishes to do to me. I have a particular image in my mind which arouses me greatly: a woman bound to an old kind of torture instrument. I saw this picture in a sex museum in Amsterdam. The woman is unable to move, even slightly. She is bound securely to a steel trestle by her neck, hands and feet. (This steel trestle is difficult to describe. You should see it – it's so gorgeous!) Of course, in my fantasy I am the woman strapped to that torture instrument and my partner is licking my clitoris until I have an orgasm. I can feel everything but am powerless to move.

Charlotte, 20, Sales Executive
I fantasise that I'm an interior designer and I'm working for a rich, good-looking bachelor. I've been told that I'm not allowed to go into one of the rooms in the house I'm decorating. But curiosity gets the better of me. I enter the forbidden room and find all sorts of sexual aids and toys. I'm examining some straps that are hanging from the ceiling and draping on the floor

when my employer enters the room, closes the door behind him and locks it. Startled, I turn round to find I've been caught. I try to speak and give some explanation as to why I'm there but he raises his finger to his mouth, gesturing me to be quiet. I can see anger in his face but his eyes glisten with excitement.

He orders me to strip and I stand frozen to the spot, wondering if he's serious. When I don't move, he pulls on a tassel hanging from the ceiling by the door. A distant bell can be heard. Another door opens – one I had not noticed previously – and three men enter, wearing masks and little else. The bachelor gestures to them and they surround me like bees around honey. The men start to undress me. At first I feel I should protest, but the look on the bachelor's face makes me think otherwise. Although he tries to hide his anticipation, a strong sturdy movement in his trousers gives him away. Before I realise it, the men have me stripped naked and are starting to tie me into the straps. My wrists and ankles are bound, a support is fastened tightly around my waist, straps are placed around my thighs and buttocks and a collar is put around my neck with the lead hooked to the ceiling.

The three men step back, allowing the bachelor to walk slowly around me, examining every inch of my exposed body. Although his hands never touch me, I can feel the heat of his eyes piercing my skin. I look at the three men; their cocks are visible through the material. Just as I think the inspection will go on for ever, the bachelor steps back. He orders the men to make me ready and one of them steps towards me. He whispers in my ear that he's going to enjoy this and takes one of my breasts in his hand. He rolls my nipple, pinching it hard; the pain is surprisingly pleasurable. He lowers his head and starts sucking and biting the hardened flesh. Another of the men moves closer and starts to work on my other breast, squeezing and sucking gently. The heat rises between my legs and it feels as though I could heat the entire room. The third man pulls on the cords hanging from the ceiling, forcing my legs up and open, exposing my private place for all to see.

The third man smiles and buries his fingers deep inside me; my juices are running down them. He licks them clean. He kneels in front of me and pushes his face between my legs, licking and probing me with his tongue. My eyes close in enjoyment. I don't know which man is going to give me the most pleasure: the first, roughly handing my breast and nipple; the second, caressing and sucking gently; or the third, his head buried deep between my legs, flicking his tongue quickly but gently over my clitoris while probing inside me with his fingers.

I can feel myself getting hotter and hotter until I can do nothing but let them bring me to my peak. The man between my legs laps up my come and then whispers in my ear that I taste good. The men step away from me and move to the other side of the room. One of the men bends another over and penetrates him from behind while the third circles to the front to accept his mouth around his manhood. Watching the men give each other pleasure keeps the heat glowing between my legs.

The bachelor undoes his zip and pulls out his manhood from his trousers. Big and proud, a bead of glistening moisture runs down to the base. He enters me with ease and pumps me with rhythmic strokes. He thrusts harder and harder inside me, then faster and faster. I hear a cry of pleasure and open my eyes to see that the three men are climaxing. As I watch the men's enjoyment, I feel my own reaching its heights. One final push deep inside me and we both climax together.

Everyone straightens up and the three men leave the

room. The bachelor kisses me softly on the lips and whispers, 'Thank you.' I never do know which colours I pick for the interior design.

Sandra, 35, Civil Servant
I think about myself being dominated, in bondage or being a sex slave. I find the idea of nipple and clitoris piercing a turn-on; also sensory deprivation and bondage pictures or stories. I think about being teased, put in restraints, blindfolded with a penis gag and thrown into a room full of men who will fondle me.

My fantasy is having my breasts bound by a dominant male and being made to put on a soft, opaque PVC mac. I would be taken out with just that on; naked underneath, but with thumb cuffs. I would be led to a car and told to sit in the passenger seat. My hands would be tied behind the seat. The seat would be reclined. My legs would be tied apart: one to the gearstick, the other to the door handle. I would be driven around with the man fondling my bound breasts through the PVC mac, or teasing my clitoris.

Eileen, 54, Retired Clerical Assistant
Back in the 50s girls were much less well informed than they are today. Sex education was a thing of the future. I must have been sixteen before I explored my own body and found the entrance to my vagina. When I reached puberty and my hormones began to surge, I had a Girl Guides Diary, which gave First Aid advice about drowning. It recommended that the victim be wrapped in a blanket with a hot-water bottle placed between their legs and another at the soles of their feet. I remember finding the idea very erotic and fantasised about being rescued by a handsome man. It is hard to believe that this mild fantasy could produce the intense burning sensation between my legs, which I found very exciting but also disturbing. Being a bit of a loner,

I never discussed it with anyone and believed myself to be 'not very nice' for having such thoughts.

I grew up in a mining community and shared a staircase with our next-door neighbours. One day, when I was just beginning to mature, I had been to fill the kettle outside and, as I returned, Ken, who lived next door and was the nearest thing I had to a brother, leapt out at me. I retaliated by drenching him with water and we struggled playfully. We collapsed giggling in the middle of the living-room floor. When I recovered my breath I discovered that my blouse had burst open and Ken's hand was cupping my breast. Neither of us referred to it and we just got up and went about whatever we had been doing previously. However, I thought about it for a long time.

I have persuaded my husband to buy glamour magazines, which fire my imagination, but it makes me feel guilty. I feel I must be abnormal for wanting to look at this kind of material as the articles are sleazy and degrading to women.

My favourite fantasy began as an erotic dream, which I extended when I woke up. I'm alone in a bar, feeling tired, dejected and unloved. A stranger enters and comes directly towards me and sits at my table. He responds immediately to my mood, strokes my knee under the table, and whispers that he knows just what I need to make me feel better. He is tall and slender with long, tapering fingers, and he repeatedly smooths back his fair hair, which keeps falling over his face.

He pleads with me to allow him to heal me and eventually I agree to go with him. Outside it is snowing and growing dark. He tucks my hand under his arm and guides me through the darkening city streets. When we arrive at a tall, Victorian house he unlocks the door and ushers me inside. The house is in darkness, but he doesn't switch on any lights. Instead, he guides me up a staircase until we reach the attic floor.

Here, he turns on a light and I am surprised to find that it's warm and comfortable with stripped-pine floors strewn with brightly coloured cushions. One wall is made entirely of glass and, through the swirling snowflakes, across the rooftops, I can see the distant lights of the city. The house is silent and I feel remote and distanced from the outside world. The stranger comes to stand beside me, and then white gauze curtains swing across the expanse of glass, shutting out the light.

He draws me into the room, smoothing back my hair, and tells me to undress. I feel self-conscious but obey. He sits watching me, fully clothed, a beatific smile curving his lips. He pours two goblets of wine and hands one to me.

He reaches for my hands and I watch in fascination as he binds leather straps around my wrists. Then I am on my feet with my arms extended upwards, suspended from a sturdy hook secured with a roof truss. I am not afraid, even though I have difficulty keeping my feet in contact with the floor. My body is stretched to its utmost, my muscles already aching from the strain, and yet I long for him to touch me and want to feel his hands roving over me. Instead, he moves out of my line of vision to somewhere behind me, and I am left swaying gently on my hook.

When he returns he has removed his shirt, and I notice for the first time that he is wearing soft, black leather trousers that mould themselves to his slim hips and well-shaped legs. He holds a riding crop and a long peacock feather. I lick my lips, which have gone suddenly dry, and I feel my nipples spring to tingling erection as I contemplate the whip. He advances towards me and taps my jutting pubis with the tip of the whip. I gasp, feeling a sudden rush of moisture between my thighs, and he smiles his enigmatic smile in acknowledgement of my growing excitement. Without warning he delivers a stinging blow across both cheeks of my bare bottom and I squeal in surprise and confusion. Several more follow the first; not excessively painful, but hard enough to sting and have me bouncing wildly on the end of my hook. These are followed by the feather being trailed lightly over my skin, paying particular attention to my most sensitive areas and bringing on a quivering arousal. Twice more he alternates the whip and the feather and I am covered in perspiration. When he lowers me to the floor I reach for him earnestly, but he presses me backwards and secures my wrist restraints to the attachments on the skirting board. He laughs when I part my legs invitingly, but reaches for a jug and drizzles a thick stream of stickiness all over me.

His eyes are bright with anticipation as he prepares to lick me clean. I writhe in ecstasy when his tongue flicks delicately over the tips of my nipples, before drawing each of them in turn into his mouth and sucking them enthusiastically. Leisurely he works his way down over my belly, slurping noisily until he reaches my crotch, and I begin to hyperventilate as I feel his tongue slide between my sex lips in search of my throbbing clitoris. Mercilessly, he lashes me to a frenzy until, at last, as I lie limp and breathless, he unzips his trousers and releases a penis of substantial proportions, which juts aggressively at a right angle to his body. He stands over me for several moments, allowing me time to appreciate it before spreading me open and driving its considerable length inside me.

Sometime later I find myself back at the wine bar with no clear recollection of how I got there. My mood is one of blissful euphoria. My bottom still burns from the kiss of the whip and the rest of me glows with the memory of his other attentions. I look up and see the stranger entering the bar. He raises one eyebrow and smiles enigmatically as he passes my table, before joining a redhead on the other side of the room. I glance at my watch as I prepare to leave and am amazed to discover that a mere half-hour has elapsed since I first arrived. Later that night, as I prepare for bed, I discover that I am not wearing any knickers and, though I search for them, I am not able to find them.

Gayle, 39, Manageress

I think about bondage and being dominated by very strong-minded men and women. I think about being fucked by two or three women at a time while a man watches, or by two women and two men, possibly using machinery.

My fantasy begins with me and my husband buying a cottage. There is an attic, and one day I find some old journals written by a woman called Lilli. One journal tells of a cellar room under the cottage, full of weird and wonderful gadgets. One day I go exploring to look for this room. I locate it behind the racks in the wine cellar. I go in and I find it is just as Lilli described: there are rows of beds fitted with different pieces of strange equipment. A door opens to the right and this woman comes and stands next to me and starts to explain the function of the various pieces of equipment. There is a bust massager to enhance the breasts, a spanking machine, and a hood that can detect exactly what turns you on. There is also a rocking horse that holds a vibrator. The woman turns out to be the keeper of the room, and two or three times a week I visit the room and use the equipment.

Eleanor, 40, Social Services

I think about being spanked, punished and, yes, raped. It has always been spanking that has done it for me. I can remember reading a story about it when I was very young and being fascinated. I think about rough, rugged macho men such as cowboys and builders; feeling powerless so a man can do anything he wanted with you. I imagine being the only female in a totally male environment.

My fantasy is written out as a short sexy story.

The ranch was completely silent as the girl crept downstairs, one hand gripping the rail. Her heart was thudding and her mouth had the dry feeling of terror, which made her swallow and try to salivate. She shivered in the thin nightshirt and padded on towards her uncle's study. Opening the door she was relieved to see the familiar humped shape of him under his blankets on the makeshift bed. He turned suddenly and leant up on one elbow. His voice was alert and he looked wide awake.

'Becky, what the hell—?'

The girl closed the door. 'I've had a bad dream and I'm cold,' she said. 'Can I climb in with you?'

He paused for a moment and then pulled the bed-clothes back. 'Jump in and be quick about it. This is a man's rest you're disturbing.'

She clambered in the big lumpy bed. Her uncle had already turned his back on her to go back to sleep. She snuggled in the warmth of his back and the masculine scent of him was evident. Tentatively she stretched up against him through her thin nightshirt.

Gil Favour was uneasy. Becky was gorgeous and totally unaware of the effect she had on men. She was twenty and he had to keep reminding her not to sashay around in her nightclothes when the ranch hands were around. Gil was not her real uncle but she'd always called him Uncle Gil. She sighed and pulled herself even closer, her hand brushing against his cock. She drew back.

'What's that?' she asked.

He smiled. 'It's a cock, Becky, and a very stiff one at that,' he said.

She pressed her mouth into his shoulder and there was a short silence. She shivered. 'Can I touch it, please?' she asked. She reached out a small hand to grab the hot wand of flesh. He groaned, and it was as much as he could do not to come there and then.

'Oh,' she breathed innocently. 'It feels lovely. It's warm, but why is it so hard and big? Oh, I want to see it, Uncle Gil, please.'

It was time she learnt, he thought. He rolled on to his back and drew the covers down. Her mouth opened wide in amazement.

'It's huge!' She looked at him with big eyes and whispered, 'Is it true what a man does to a woman with that? One of the cowboys told me they poke it inside you.'

'I think it's time a man showed you the pleasures of loving before one of those young boys spoils your dreams,' said Gil. He took hold of her bottom firmly and pulled her hips towards him so she could feel the strength of his erection pressing into her lower belly. Then he moved his hand to the front and rubbed her mound through her knickers. She put her hand out to stop him. He nuzzled her ear.

'Now, don't you tell me you don't do this to yourself in bed at night and then get a nice feeling. Well, now you'll find it even better when a man does it for you.'

She buried her face in his shoulder. He lifted her chin. 'Look at me,' he said, and when those delectable lips came up, he kissed her, all the while his rubbing becoming stronger and more insistent. His fingers slid into her knickers and found the little nub of pleasure. While his thumb rubbed gently on that, his fingers explored the hot wet opening and found her wet – so wet. Her hips rose and fell, imitating the sex act she hadn't yet experienced. He breathed against her ear.

'I have to take your pants down so you can open

your legs wide for me.' He started to tug at the cotton material.

Becky began to panic. 'No, stop, I don't want you to,' she cried, but his heavy muscular body lay across her, pinning her arms to the bed while his hand continued to rip her pants down. She was struggling and wriggling under him now. He lifted her nightshirt, exposing her jutting breasts. Lowering his mouth to them he sucked at the brown tips, drawing a small cry of pleasure from her. He lifted his head and let his gaze wander the length of her body, all the while stroking her soft skin and pulling her thighs apart so he could examine the thing she was denying him.

Becky could have died with embarrassment; no man had ever seen her naked and she felt the heat flood into her cheeks. He put his hand on the inside of her thigh.

'Open your legs for me.'

'No.' She clamped her legs firmly together, trapping his hand.

'Don't play hard to get, Becky,' he said, ''cos one way or another you're going to get fucked tonight, whether you like it or not. It's high time you learnt about loving from a man.'

Her face crumpled. She started to cry but he ignored her tears and prised her legs apart, settling himself on top of her. Taking hold of his cock, he felt around for the entrance. God, she was tight! His fingers splayed the opening wide enough for him to get the tip in and, once it was in, it was an easy job to thrust into her right to the hilt, but he forced himself to slow down and only go in a small way.

'Stop it, Uncle Gil. Stop it, it's hurting me. I don't want to,' Becky protested.

Suddenly he lost patience. Getting off her, he dragged her to the armchair and threw her across an arm. Raising her nightshirt, he slapped her bare bottom hard again and again. Already sore from an earlier spanking at the hands of Gil, she answered to his immediate authority.

'Get your legs apart when I tell you, and stick your bottom out,' he ordered. Grasping her hips, he lifted her up towards him and rammed himself hard into her and started thrusting in and out. Her hand came back to push futilely against his groin.

'Oh, stop, Uncle Gil,' she said. 'Please stop. I don't like it.'

He grasped her wrist and held it firmly against her lower back. 'Becky, honey, you are really tight because it's your first time. You have to stop struggling and relax.'

She stopped struggling and, in a small voice, said, 'I'm sorry. I'll do as you say. I want you to show me.'

He withdrew and pulled her up and gathered her in his arms. 'That's better. Now, let's start again,' he said. Taking hold of her hand he led her back to the bed. He sat down naked and Becky stood before him. 'First lesson. When a man needs a woman he wants to see what he's going to get, so take your nightdress off so I can see you.'

She squirmed with embarrassment. Meeting his eyes, she grasped the hem of the thin cotton gown and drew it up slowly. Gil watched the long slim legs appear and the rounded hips with the vee of brown curly hair, the indentation of her waist, her rounded high breasts crested with brown nipples. She let her nightshirt drop to the floor. Her face was crimson and she shuddered as she stood before him completely naked. Gil let his gaze wander from toe to head, taking in her loveliness.

'Now turn around,' he said.

She nervously turned around, not taking her eyes from his face until her back was towards him. He looked at her reddened bottom and a slight smile played across his lips. Pulling her back towards him he sat her on his knee and the feeling of her flesh against his brought back the urge more strongly. He felt her pussy; it was soaking. This time it would be easy. He pushed her back on to the bed and said urgently, 'Now open your legs really wide for me.'

This time she let her legs fall apart willingly and he entered her quickly. Grasping her bottom he pulled her up towards him and thrust hard. Her mouth opened with a wide 'Oh' and then she relaxed and her hips moved up to meet his. It only took a few minutes of this before his head went back and he came inside her. He rested his head on her shoulder.

'Now do as you're told next time and you'll enjoy it.'

Annabelle, 29, Civil Servant

The general themes running through my favourite fantasies are of being overpowered and seduced roughly by one or more people; also, being beaten and raped and being tied up and helpless. Alternatively, beating a man (or occasionally a woman) in public and then fucking them. Bondage turns me on and I write for a bisexual magazine called *The Chain Letter* which makes me horny. I also show interested guests our 'toy' collection. I like group sex and public sex as well as public SM. I love my long leather boots and my partner's corset. I loved the agony of having my nipples pierced – slowly, steadily and without painkillers – while I was tied down.

The Story of O was an early turn-on for me. I didn't particularly eroticise clothing, apart from a general interest in leather. When I was at boarding school, I would get very turned on by being massaged by my best friend. I would imagine that I was tied down and helpless. I would even tie myself up when I was about thirteen. Then, at sixteen, I discovered Nancy Friday.

My favourite fantasy goes like this. I've been a

naughty girl. It's never clear what I've done but I'm in trouble. My male partner is angry and decides to make an example of me. We have a dinner party that evening and, as the meal ends, he suddenly tells me to take my clothes off. The other guests, of course, look horrified, and my partner reassures them that there is no problem and that I have misbehaved and have to be punished.

Once I am naked he bends me over a chair. It hurts, and my back is taut and stretched. The other guests clearly don't know where to look and are stunned and silent. Suddenly my whole being is suffused with pain as a cane is forced, at high speed, into the crease of my arse. I stiffen and try to move. That brings another stroke, then another. I am whimpering, crying out with each blow. The other guests are forgotten as all I can do is try to survive the caning. Suddenly I realise it's finished. The pain is slowly ebbing away.

Before I can take in what's happening, I feel cool grease being forced up the entrance to my arse. I wriggle, trying to get away. It doesn't work; I am being firmly held down. Opening my eyes, I see our guests; many of them are openly waiting, particularly the men. Suddenly my arse is entered roughly. A hand clamps over my mouth to prevent me from swearing. My partner thrusts into me over and over again. Each push feels as if it is splitting my body apart and brings me closer to the brink of orgasm. A final thrust, and then I feel myself full of hot come and he falls on top of me. Another man takes his place. At this point the fantasy tends to have fulfilled its purpose.

Tina, 35, Clerical Assistant
Male domination is my thing; also, being spanked. I can't understand why this is, as I've never allowed men to dominate me in everyday life. However, I love to be dominated sexually. I love the thought of people

in authority taking advantage of me, but only sexually! I love men in uniform, especially policemen. After a work out at the gym I could rip the clothes off the first police officer I bump into!

This is the fantasy I think about when I'm out walking during the summer months. I always feel very aroused when I walk about in the sun. No one is around, so I take my T-shirt off. I can feel the breeze on my body. It feels so good that I decide to let the air get to my breasts. I pull the front of my bra down so they are still supported but fully exposed. I start to play with them as I walk. I lick my fingers and gently rub the wet over my nipples. I feel the wetness between my legs and I look around and see that nobody is about. I lay my T-shirt on the ground and sit down and pull my shorts down so I can relieve the throbbing between my legs. While I am squeezing my tits and probing my fingers deep into me and stimulating my clit, I don't realise that I am being watched. Once I have screamed out with my orgasm I open my eyes to see this man (he is always about 50 years old) standing over me, looking really angry. He starts telling me how I should be ashamed of myself. When I say that I'm not, he tells me that he is going to teach me a lesson I won't forget. He then grabs hold of my wrist and pulls me to my feet. He takes me to a tree stump that is lying just behind us, sits down, puts me across his knee, pulls down my shorts and starts to give me a good spanking.

My arse is on fire, and he slides his hand between my legs and can feel how turned on I am by what he is doing. He tells me how bad I am and that I need to feel his belt. He bends me over the tree with my bare arse exposed and hot. The breeze adds to the pleasure. He slowly removes his belt and after about six lashes across my bare arse he drops his trousers and fucks me hard from behind. I still don't know who he is and never find out.

I would like to see a disciplinarian a couple of times a week, then, while my arse is still hot, be fucked by my boyfriend.

Shelly, 35, Chef

I have several recurring elements in my fantasies. They are: being spanked by an older man or younger woman; being made love to by two men anally and vaginally at the same time; bondage; voyeurism – being watched, but pretending not to know. When I was young, my parents used to have sex magazines. I loved reading all the naughty stories, so I grew up in a very sexy household; very open. I remember one book in particular, which was in Italian; a cartoon of a young girl who falls asleep on a beach. She is dreaming of sex and is woken up by about fifteen young men who all fuck her in as many ways as you can imagine. In the end, they come all over her body and in her mouth until she's covered in it. I had my first orgasm with that book. I imagined she was me. I wished for years for something like that to happen to me.

Reading erotica never fails to turn me on. I am now into body piercing. I have my tongue, belly-button and nipples pierced, and have some tattoo bracelets on my upper arms. I find tattooed and pierced people sexy, especially bikers. I am a biker myself. When you get a few hundred bikers at a party, the sexuality in the air is intense! I love sexy talk, flirting in groups when everyone is on a natural high and buzzing.

Here's my favourite fantasy. It's an evening with good wine flowing. Myself, two men and one other woman. The girl is laid on her back and I'm licking her clit while I'm being fucked by one of the men. The other has his cock in her mouth. The girl puts on a strap-on dildo and fucks me, while one man is screwing my ass. The other then puts his cock in my mouth. The men decide we have been bad so set about giving us the spanking of our lives. We are facing each other across their laps and we kiss, tongues deep in each other's mouths. Then they make us 69 and finger-fuck each other while they watch in close-up. The men tie us up then blindfold us, taking it in turn to fuck us alternately. The room goes silent. We cannot see but we feel the men come on us: in our mouths, on our hair and breasts. They untie her and put her on top of me. Then we are tied together in the 69 position and are spanked by hand and by a cruel whippy stick till we are begging to stop.

All the time this is happening, they force us to continue licking each other. We are then untied. They lie on their backs and we are made to sit in them and pump them until they nearly come. They stop at the last minute then we sit on their faces and make them lick, suck and nibble until we orgasm out little hearts out. We turn them over then out comes the whippy stick and we take it in turns to whip them. The girl sucks and pinches my nipples then once again she fucks me with the strap-on while the men watch, helpless. We finish the evening with everyone giving me a very messy oily massage.

Tracey-Jay, 28, Electronic Motor Assembler
The recurring themes in my sexual fantasies are of bondage and light S&M. I arrive home from work before my husband and decide to treat him. Going upstairs, I shower then dress in sexy black underwear, suspenders and stockings. I then lie on the bed to wait for him. He arrives home and, seeing me lying on the bed, he decides to punish me. He gets five scarves out of my drawer and ties my hands and feet to the bedposts. He undresses to reveal his immense erection

and blindfolds me with the fifth scarf. Then the fun begins.

He begins by kissing my arms, legs, neck and stomach all over, carefully avoiding my bust and fanny. He carries on until I have to beg him to kiss me more intimately. He gently kisses my bust with light, delicate kisses and, every so often, licks my nipples until they are erect and standing up proudly. Then he begins on my fanny, covering it with light kisses and starting to investigate further with his tongue. Now he starts to get rougher, tormenting my clit by alternatively licking and sucking it. I can't stand it any more and beg him to fuck me, but he continues to torment my clit. Eventually I experience a huge climax and, before my body can recover, he is fucking me. My body is racked with repeated mini-orgasms and my fanny is soaked. At last I feel his own release within me. Then – and only then – does he release me from my bonds and blindfold. The deprivation of my senses makes my orgasm extremely intense, and we both fall into a blissful sleep in each other's arms.

Shelagh, 18, Fitness Trainer
I think a lot about making love in a barn or on a haystack, or being tied up and blindfolded and being spoon-fed stuff from the fridge. My fantasy begins as a normal night out; just two of us going for a meal and a drink, passing the odd dirty remark and gradually getting more turned on. We get a bit tipsy and head home. We sit down on the settee, having a glass of wine, and then he starts to kiss and touch me. He takes off my clothes and then his. He blindfolds me and leads me into the kitchen and ties me up. I feel a cold chill and my nipples get even harder. He sits me on the floor and tells me to open my mouth. He puts a spoon in my mouth with what tastes like yoghurt on it. He puts some more in my mouth and it drops down

my cleavage. He licks it off. Next, I feel an ice cube; he is rubbing it around my lips, my neck, and now my cleavage. He carries on experimenting with other foods, and then we make hot steamy love over the kitchen table.

Jenny, 31, Carer

I have always liked dominant men. In my teens I found hairy men sexy, but now I don't mind. I have a fetish for black underwear – it used to be white – and I love velvet, lace and floral scents and musk. I've been reading porn since I was fifteen.

I have mainly historical fantasies, and one favourite is that of having sex in a hay loft. This is daft, as I have hay fever in real life! I quite like actors such as Colin Firth, Sean Bean, Kenneth Brannagh and Mel Gibson. All my life I have loved history, especially the sixteenth century. It sounds corny, but my favourite man in history is Henry the Eighth. If I went back in time, though, I'd like to be like Moll Flanders in Defoe's infamous novel. The one thing that would improve my sex life would be a tall, red-haired, blue-eyed man, preferably Welsh and built like a rugby player!

Chapter Seven
Not Just Bodies

Without taboos, sex wouldn't seem half as naughty. The thrill of the forbidden – of going that bit further than we ought – evokes memories of childhood pranks: sneaking into places we shouldn't and making off with a trophy, however humble, and creasing with laughter afterwards at our triumph. It is about the chance of getting away with it, of defying the rules, outwitting authority and having a good time in the process. I put a lot of store in the concept of inappropriate behaviour; it is a friend of erotic fantasy and a prevalent theme in Black Lace novels. I like to remind authors of erotica that it's a lot ruder for your character to take her knickers off in the office than at an orgy. Erotic fantasies are about the unexpected; the 'what if?' Unlike dreams, where we are at the mercy of our subconscious, we can cast our players, choose our locations, dress or undress ourselves in whatever finery we choose and go as far as we like. We can visualise ourselves in eroticised situations which, in real life, we would most likely be too embarrassed to initiate.

The fantasies I have grouped into this section are,

simply, those that are about more than 'some people having sex'. They are the fantasies where subjects other than the purely physical come into play; where the human body may not be the central focus. This includes fetishism, and clothes associated with dressing for sex; bondage, spanking, punishment, ritual and all the instruments of correction; and more far-out and unusual themes, such as animals and aliens. The old-fashioned phrase would be 'kinky sex', which is a useful umbrella term, but it seems somewhat outdated in this world of high-fashion rubber parties at prestigious venues and the acceptance of fetish clothes into the couture end of the catwalk. Ten years ago there were a handful of clothes designers, retail outlets and nightclubs catering to such tastes. However, with fetish fashion stores opening in central London and many cities in the US, and no longer hiding behind concrete shopfronts and blacked-out windows; with numerous documentaries and full-colour glossy magazines covering the latest developments in the fetish world; and with more reading material (both fiction paperbacks and lavishly illustrated coffee-table books) being published about unconventional or 'non-vanilla' sex, being kinky has become a lifestyle choice to flaunt rather than to keep as a guilty secret.

Doctors, Nurses and Other Uniforms

Whereas men tend to focus on visualising their ideal partner's perfect body parts, women veer towards imagining situations where character dynamics are at work. This is nowhere better illustrated than in the fantasies that transgress the boundaries of rank or social convention. This can be a potent aphrodisiac; from making advances to a complete stranger to stripping for the doctor just that bit too provocatively. Now that we are adults and the prize for 'getting away with it' is sexual conquest with someone we shouldn't be doing rude things with, the stakes are higher. If we did make a pass at our doctor and he refused, not only would we be caught out being filthy, we would be so embarrassed by our behaviour that we'd never be able to look him in the eye again. That's why many of the fantasies in the first section are about the other party taking control; we don't have to be shamed into having to ask for what we really want. Rank and profession are fetishised in these fantasies in a way where the person's occupation is usually concerned with taking charge. By putting ourselves in the care of another, we are surrendering responsibility. We have to trust our dentist; s/he has the means to cause us a lot of pain. We also have to do what s/he says. This goes, too, for the police, for firefighters; for anyone whose occupation requires our complicity for them to be able to do their job properly – even traffic wardens.

How many women go weak at the thought of a good-looking doctor, complete with his white coat and clean hands, wanting to make a thorough examination of us? No wonder the US television series *ER* was an instant hit; whoever cast George Clooney as Doctor Ross knew a thing or two about the appeal of medical fantasies. The other side of the coin is the ever-popular male fantasy of the sexy nurse. Good-looking, womanly, caring and naughty, she will make our stay in hospital memorable in the best way possible. The medical scenario appeals to both sexes as we often want the responsibility for our sexual desires to be taken away from us and put into the hands of those who are well equipped to deal with our needs. The environment is clean and the equipment is easily fetishised – all that rubber, those tubes, the snappy gloves and probing devices.

It isn't a huge leap for the imagination to take the medical paraphernalia to a sexual level: making those uniforms a bit too tight, a bit more shiny; and those stethoscopes a bit more bendy and phallic. The first fantasy in this section is an elaborate dentist fantasy. Ever since seeing Steve Martin leap around as the sadistic dentist in *Little Shop of Horrors*, I've seen the appeal of this particular occupation fetish. The forcing open of the mouth, the probing inside; it's a crude reworking of the basic sex act, but it's his power and her vulnerability that are the determining factors here, not the pain or the process of actually having teeth drilled. Most medical fantasies are a world away from medical reality and are not about pain at all. It's not the teeth that are important, it's the powerlessness at the hands of a fetishised dominant other.

Police and firemen are also on this list. Some of the women I've spoken to actually admitted to hanging around fire stations and flirting outrageously in the hope that they got lucky. Every time I asked what was the overriding important factor, they said it was the uniform. One woman actually began an affair with a fireman after visiting him at his station. When he turned up at her house in his everyday street clothes she lost interest. If only the poor lass had been brave enough to tell him what it really was she wanted.

This is why dressing up can be so much fun. If your lover has a thing for traffic wardens, put on that flat cap and get very stern with him. You'll be rewarded with an enthusiasm that only a large dose of Viagra could match. It is worth remembering that most of us – men and women – are shy when it comes to taking the lead and tend towards being the submissive party. Few of us want to run the risk of being sexually dominant; it means that you have to work that much harder, always thinking ahead to what scenario you are going to initiate and which paraphernalia has to be on hand.

The fantasies in this section are meticulous; where a

particular material or object is given emphasis, every
detail is lovingly recorded. In Eve's fantasy it isn't any
old drill that her dentist wields; it's a drill with a long
handle made of black anodised aluminium. Her
appointment card has gilt edging with gold lettering
and the surgery is in one of the most exclusive areas in
the city. Everything is stylised to perfection in the
medical fantasy.

Eve, 32, Doctor
The recurring themes in my fantasies are dental surger-
ies, bondage in a four-poster bed or being trapped in
snow in a remote cottage. My favourite turn-ons now
are definitely medical or dental examinations and Black
Lace books.

Here is my fantasy: an unexpected dental appointment arrives in the post. Its style resembles a sumptu-
ous invitation card with gilt edging and gold lettering.
It requests the pleasure of my company at the surgery
and the appointment is in the evening. The address of
the surgery is in one of the exclusive areas of town. I
choose my sexiest underwear and a black button-
through dress.

I arrive at the surgery and a male voice comes
through the entry-phone speaker and invites me to
take a seat in the waiting room at the top of the stairs.
The waiting room is luxurious with a large fireplace
and an ornate gilt mirror above it. I hang up my coat
and take a seat and wait. After what seems like an age
a voice calls out, 'Good evening, Miss [name]. Please
come through to the surgery. I will be with you in a
moment.'

Moving through into the surgery, I see a white
leather dental chair with an overhead light and the
usual instrument consoles and trays beside the chair.
The room is dimly lit and the chair is picked out by the
overhead light. I walk over and gingerly sit on the

chair, which slowly reclines. It feels comfortable, although the overhead light is dazzling in my eyes. There is a long wait and then I hear the sound of approaching footsteps. The dentist walks into the room and sits on a stool behind the head of the chair. I cannot see him. I see his arms reaching forward to adjust the light. They are strong arms covered with downy blond hairs and he has long, slender fingers. I extend my neck to see his face. He is tanned with blond hair and blue eyes. He smiles but no words are exchanged.

He secures my wrists to the armrests using soft leather straps. Although my wrists are held securely I know I could pull them free if I wanted to. As he secures a tissue under my chin his arm brushes my erect nipples. There then follows a long dental examination as he gently probes every crevice. The examination is painless and thorough, and the intimate examination of my mouth is somehow penetrative and erotic. After a pause he announces that I need some minor treatment. I simply nod; nothing needs to be said. He fits a nasal mask in place and turns on the gas. He reassures me that the gas will produce a relaxed dreamy sensation and will not put me to sleep. A sense of wellbeing and relaxation comes over me and any desire I have to resist ebbs away.

Slowly he starts to undo the buttons of my dress. After undoing each button he pauses to look into my eyes. When he has undone the last button he pulls my dress apart and stares at my breasts through the lace, then pinches one nipple. He pulls the material down to free both breasts. He takes a tube of gel from the instrument tray and squeezes a cold blob on to each breast. He then massages the gel in small circles. The jelly feels cold and tingles on my skin. Next, he reaches over to his instrument console and removes a long white tubular sucker, which he holds over each nipple in turn, drawing a cooling stream of air over the sensitive skin. Finally he sucks the gel off the skin, trapping my nipple momentarily in the end of the sucker; he pulls it free with a faint plop. Then he replaces the sucker and pulls his instrument tray nearer to the chair. My eyes are drawn to a pair of nipple clamps joined by a short chain. He attaches one to each nipple. I am aware of an initial discomfort, which fades and gives way to increasing arousal. He then pulls the dribble bib back round to cover my breasts. The rubbery plastic sticks slightly where the remains of the gel lie. The clasps are visible through the translucent material.

My black suede high heels are removed and thrown to a corner of the room. He kisses the skin between my black hold-up stockings and the lace edging of my knickers, starting on the outside and working onwards towards the tender skin on the inside of my thighs. Then he kisses the satin strip over my vulva. He inhales deeply, smelling the musky scent of my sex. My fingers stretch out and my wrists strain at the leather bonds. 'You must be patient,' he says, smiling as he looks into my eyes. He then begins to stroke my sex lips through the satin and pushes his finger in as far as the material will allow. His fingers move under the elasticated waistband. I arch my back slightly and he pulls my knickers down. They are removed in one smooth operation.

Next I feel my legs being spread so that my feet hang over the edge of the reclining chair. My right ankle is placed in a stirrup at the side of the chair and I hear the castors of the chair move around to the other side in order to attend to my other ankle, which is similarly trapped. I am bound, shamelessly exposed and exquisitely vulnerable, with my knees bent and forced apart and my most private parts exposed to his penetrating gaze.

The drills above me hang like predators over their prey with the coiled hoses hanging down almost touching me between the legs. He pulls a large drill from its holder and gently spreads my sex lips with one hand to expose my engorged clitoris. The drill has a long handle made of black anodised aluminium, and at the end there is a small polished silver T-piece. From one end a pointed drill bit protrudes but the opposite end is rounded and smooth and altogether less menacing. He holds the rounded end so it just touches my now aching bud. He presses the pedal with his foot; the air turbine bursts into life and the drill begins its high-speed rotation. The whining noise would normally reduce me to a nervous wreck but I feel relaxed and welcome his attentions. As the drill bit spins harmlessly in the air it sends out a fine cooling spray of water, which settles like dew on the inside of my thighs and on the hairs of my sex. The turbine transmits its exquisite vibrations and sends waves of pleasure as he begins to circle my clitoris slowly. I can feel my juices trickling down, mixing with the spray from the drill. I sigh softly and press my feet into the stirrups, grinding my vulva on to the wickedly vibrating cold metal of his handpiece. He stops and replaces the drill in its holder.

His finger gently circles the skin of my outer lips and he inserts one then two fingers into my vagina, observing that I am wet. He smiles knowingly to himself. Next he reaches over to the cupboard behind the chair and removes a blue plastic butterfly-shaped object. As he turns it over in the beam of his operating light, I see that one side has numerous fine rubbery spines and black straps hanging from each corner. On the side opposite the spines there is a black cylinder and, leading from the cylinder to the instrument tray, is a coiled hose. The dentist, seeing my direction of gaze, says, 'The compressed air does not only power the turbines of the drills. When I press the foot pedal the spines on the butterfly will wiggle and twist just where you most like to be touched. The harder I press the pedal, the more power I will deliver, and the more stimulation you will get. You'll get pleasure where you most need it and you won't feel a thing – in your mouth, that is.'

Moving slowly and deliberately he places the butterfly over my vulva. I lift my buttocks off the chair, enabling him to thread the straps under me. He pulls the buckle tight and I feel the soft spines invading my swollen lips, ready to begin their delicious assault on my clitoris. 'Open your mouth now, please,' he says. In my aroused state I feel no anxiety; none of the usual butterflies in the stomach. I open my mouth to his inspection. He places a hook-shaped sucker over my bottom lip and, with his little finger, gently pulls the corner of my mouth downwards and sideways, inserting a dental roll between my lips and gums. Now I am effectively stripped, gagged and bound in a compromising position by a complete stranger.

I lie back and wait for the treatment to begin. First the mirror is inserted into my mouth. There is a momentary pause and then the high-pitched whine of the drill starts inside my mouth. I am barely aware of the dental treatment as the spines of the vibrating butterfly twist, turn and insinuate themselves into my most sensitive crevice. The treatment passes in an erotic haze of pleasure. There is no pain and all sensation is concentrated on my sex.

After an indeterminate length of time I wake up in the chair with my clothes in disarray but my legs and hands free from the restraints. The dentist is no longer in the room but there is another appointment card propped up on the instrument tray. My nipples still feel slightly sore from the clamps. I pick up my clothes and dress slowly. I return to the waiting room to pick up my coat and pocket the appointment card. This is one dentist's appointment I will be sure to keep.

Clare, 38, Freelance Designer

I've always had an active imagination – sexually and otherwise – although I never had an orgasm until I was seventeen. I had been having sex since I was fourteen but didn't know about the clitoris until three years later. Sometimes I find it difficult to choose a viewpoint when having a fantasy. Sometimes I'm watching the entire scene and am not directly involved; sometimes I'm the man, fucking the woman; sometimes I'm two people, so I can be both male and female. However, there has to be a cock involved – or several men wanking. It is always male masturbation that does it for me, rather than imagining being fucked. I think this is because I was totally fascinated with male genitals after seeing a man expose himself to me when I was quite young. Far from being frightened, I was curious and stood staring in amazement until the guy had finished. He must have thought it was his lucky day!

I'm waiting to see a doctor in a squeaky clean, modernist environment. Not at all like an NHS hospital but more like a building in a futurist vision. There's nothing seriously wrong with me but my minor complaint requires an internal examination. When I'm finally taken to a cubicle, the only doctor who is able to examine me is one who has previously been found guilty of improper conduct and now works as a manager. He is not usually allowed to touch the female patients but they are under-staffed and they make an exception just this once.

We are alone in the white room. He comes in with his white coat on. He stretches across me to get at his instruments and I can already feel he has a massive boner under his tunic. He is good-looking and has nice

173

thick hair and glasses. He looks very unassuming and not at all like the pervert he really is. He asks me to strip off and, when I'm down to my underwear (rubber knickers, stockings and a very tight top), he takes time to look at me, rubbing his groin and whispering that he's going to make my inspection enjoyable – if not for me, then certainly for him. He orders me to lie on my front. He pulls my knickers down, gets a handful of greasy substance and rubs it along the crease of my bottom. He then starts telling me how hard he is and that I'm going to be begging for it within five minutes. He kneels on the bed behind me and rubs himself up against my greasy hole. My cunt is begging to be filled by his thick cock, although I also want to take it in my mouth. He gets it out and tells me that he has to release it or he will come in his pants.

Then he calls out for his helper. She is dressed up in a shiny turquoise and white PVC nurses' outfit and is exactly the kind of woman I'd really like to have sex with. Not all tepid and romantic but a filthy-minded, feisty and very intelligent woman. She has bright red hair – thick and wavy – in bunches and is pierced and tattooed and up for anything. She sits astride the bed at the pillow end and orders me to lick her through her PVC panties. I rub my tongue along the plastic while she fondles my tits and rubs her hands all over me. Then the two of them start getting it together and I'm beside myself with lust and frustration. The male doctor makes me and her writhe up against each other. I like grabbing her arse, snogging her and rubbing her between her legs. She is very responsive and is as desperate for cock as I am. He is wanking himself watching us while we rub each other. He's telling us how he can have both of us. I imagine various combinations: me fucking her with a strap-on dildo while she sucks him off; him holding her while she pretends it's against her will and I 'rape' her with my false cock, holding my hand over her mouth and being rough with her. She loves it, really. Then the best part is when he gets her to roll a condom over him and he slowly fucks me in the arse, constantly telling me how tight it is, how hard he's going to come and how much spunk is going to shoot out of his cock, etc. While he fills my tight hole, I watch her rubbing herself off, writhing all over the place before we all come together. Sometimes I think about the nurse peeing her plastic pants and getting punished – by both me and the doctor – or watching her stick dildos into her arse and cunt, getting really nasty and filthy.

Leeanne, 22, Data Inputer
I must confess I am a virgin. However, I am curious, although afraid of pregnancy and STDs, but I enjoy reading erotica. Naturally I masturbate frequently and feel I allow myself more enjoyment and exploration of my body than many women involved in sexual relationships. I am quite prepared to wait for the right man to come along before I lose my virginity. I am one of the women who read Black Lace books and think, I thought only I had fantasies like that! Men do not understand what women find erotic and this is why we must make it plain – firstly to ourselves and then to other women so they can share in this forbidden knowledge. While we may feel angered by a woman's submissiveness as written by a man, we can simply delight in its eroticism if a woman writes it. Women's erotica might be a chance for us to redeem sex and pleasure and make it something to be proud of and not ashamed of. Women being proud of their bodies can be no bad thing!

My fantasies often include men being vulnerable, leaving me in a position of power. I like the idea of a man being vulnerable due to injury and I am able to mother him; a man stripped and often whipped in front of me; or of being an FBI or a police agent so I can interrogate a man. Anything to do with riding excites me – the tight breeches, the crop, the barn full of straw. Also, men in white uniforms have a great appeal for me. The flipside is that while I am determined not to be submissive to men in reality, my fantasies are often centred around my not having control over what men do to me. Despite my general distrust of the medical profession, many fantasies centre on such matters: the lifeguard who rescues and resuscitates; the emergency room full of cute male doctors with all sorts of paraphernalia and rubber gloves.

For some reason, my favourite fantasy involves being taken to an emergency room of a large city hospital, due to an accidental or deliberate overdose/poisoning. They take my clothes off and examine me; lots of soft warm hands caress my body. Sometimes they pump my stomach. Sometimes they wear rubber gloves. Often they have to resuscitate me (mouth to mouth or by devices, by hand or by defribulator) but, of course, I am totally aware of it all, sometimes experiencing, sometimes watching it happen. Sometimes one of them will put on rubber gloves and explore inside me while others carry out various tests or treatments on my bare chest and belly.

Carole, 45, Analyst Programmer

When I was younger, I was lucky to have a lover who was a great teacher, who introduced me to much more than straight sex. Anal sex and the water bed were wonderful. He would often watch me while his friends encouraged me with words and touch. Recently, I was shaved by a lover, which was very sexy. Open-air sex is also fun and, occasionally, oral sex really stimulates me. Threesomes are brilliant. That was a fantasy which came true. I would now like to try a female lover on her own. Writing and thinking about this questionnaire is a turn-on, as are the Black Lace books, and voyeuristic fantasies.

My favourite fantasy is situated in a hospital-like environment. I like the idea of being on a medical trolley, surrounded by people – male and female – dressed in white coats. My hands and feet are immobile – I cannot see anything – but I can feel dozens of hands caressing my face, ears, neck, nipples, arms, legs, feet, stomach, labia and clitoris. They are also stimulating me with their tongues and feathers; very light touches all over my body, and each one trying to be the most erotic, to make me lose control completely. There is also somebody talking or reading about sex at the same time. A spiral, onwards and upwards, but I've yet to get to the ultimate crescendo. In this fantasy, I can tell the males from the females, and am straining to ask them for more and touch them too, but it is impossible.

Sharon, 33, Occupation Unknown
I used to get turned on by wearing certain bras and the feeling of water on my nipples making them stand out. Swimming pools and jacuzzis feature in my fantasies. I also get off on seeing a man's penis. Today I fantasise using Black Lace and romance books. I also watch X-rated movies, read *Playgirl* and get horny writing to my male pen pal. My favourite fantasy is set in a doctor's surgery, where I am lying on a table, naked. The doctor enters with only a lab coat on. He locks the door and I ask him to touch my breasts as I'm so horny. He kneads, touches and plays with my nipples. Then I feel one hand move on to my pussy. He says that I'm very moist, hot and ready for a penis to enter me. However, he first wants to put my legs up into the stirrups, so he moves me to the end of the table and then I feel him push my legs apart. Suddenly, some

fingers have entered my womanhood. He says that he wants to feel my cervix and find my G-spot.

'Please, oh please, enter your rock-hard penis into me,' I cry. I feel his hand slide out of me and a hard missile enter my pussy. He leans over to suck, lick and tongue my breasts. As he is sucking on my breasts, I can feel my cunt muscles clamping down on his penis. I tell him that I am close to climax. I want both of us to climax together. We fuck on the table many times, and then on his sofa. We suck each other in the 69 position, then fuck again. After, we take a nap, talk and touch each other until it's time to leave.

Beverley, 26, Housewife/Mother

I have recurring fantasies about men in uniform. I know a policeman and I would love him to tie me up, handcuff me and use his truncheon on me! I used to love having my ears touched a lot. It used to really get me going. If I could see a few hairs over the top of a man's shirt, it would be very nice!

I love being tied up and blindfolded – that's so mind blowing. I also like having my back kissed, and fantasise about having power over a man, so I am in control in the bedroom. I like men with long, blond hair, as long as it isn't tied back. My favourite fantasy involves being in bed with two or three men. They are giving me all their attention. They have to be big men with lots of muscles. Warrior, Trojan and Cobra from *Gladiators* would do nicely!

I love foreplay, and to have many hands and mouths all over my body would be out of this world. I love to see men go hard and I love giving blow jobs. I found that with my last partner, I often wasn't finished when he was, so having one or two men waiting in the wings would be great, as long as I call the shots. I would love this fantasy to become a reality.

Lesley, 29, Hairdresser

I have sexual fantasies several times a day. A recurring favourite is of me driving alone on the motorway. It's dark and raining and I get pulled over by two police-men. They go through the usual shit, such as asking if it's my car or not. They then both turn away from me and talk together. I am drenched from standing in the rain. One officer says that my car will have to be searched for drugs, as I fit a description of someone wanted by the police. Then they say that they will also have to search me. I struggle, so one of them handcuffs me. I'm escorted to the police car, where I sit on the back seat with the door open. They start searching me and begin to get a bit personal, rubbing my legs and groping my tits. At first they are careful, but then they get rougher. The copper who has handcuffed me makes me lie down, while the other one rips off my knickers and plunges his head between my legs. He starts kissing my cunt.

The other one has taken out his fat purple cock and makes me eat him. This goes on for a while, and then he puts his cock into my mouth and wanks hard until he comes in my mouth. He makes me swallow every drop. Just as he comes, the other copper takes out his own dick and shoves it hard into me. God, it hurts! Shit! I'm being raped by a pig, I think. He comes and comes; I feel like I'm being split in half. As they have now finished what they were doing, they turn to me and say: 'Well, madam, everything seems to be in order. Thank you for your assistance.' They take me to my car, then fuck off and leave me there, just a little bemused and sore!

Kate, 23, Sales Assistant

I tend to fantasise a few times a week. A recurring subject is lesbian sex with my boyfriend watching. I also get horny thinking about anonymous sex. I used to pleasure myself by pulling my knickers up very high so that my clitoris was stimulated. I also used to sit at my parents' bedroom window, watching a couple opposite having sex in the afternoons. I have a particular turn-on which is my boyfriend chewing the gusset of my knickers after I have worn them all day at work.

My favourite fantasy takes place when I'm alone in my bedroom. Suddenly I'm aware of someone else in the room. I look towards the door and see a very tall, broad man dressed in a US Navy officer's uniform. He has mirrored aviator sunglasses on and a peaked cap, white gloves and black patent shoes. Without a word he walks over to my bed and lifts my dress up to my waist. He tears off my knickers and climbs on to the bed. He undoes his flies, takes himself out and pushes into me. He is so big I feel I'm going to rip. He is on top of me but at arm's length. He is expressionless and I cannot see his eyes. All I can see is my reflection in his glasses.

He gets faster and faster until I explode with the most intense orgasm I have ever had. He then withdraws, puts himself away and gets off the bed and walks towards the door. Before leaving he turns back, salutes me and leaves. There is no trace of him, no smell, no taste, no bodily fluids. The only trace is in my head and the fact that my knickers have vanished.

Kinky Books, Leather Lovers, Punks and Nazis

Certain materials are considered fetishistic because of their tactile quality and associations with perverted or forbidden sex. Long thought of as the preserve of suburban English gentlemen with a penchant for mackintoshes and gas masks, rubber clothing has recently found its way into the fashion pages of style magazines. Rubber and leather have masculine connotations, as both of these fabrics were traditionally designed for industrial purposes, being hard wearing, protective and insulating. To subvert these clothes for sexual purposes (whether you are male or female) is to reject the vulnerability of human flesh in preference for feeling galvanised during the sex act; to try in some way to transmogrify ourselves into a being with special powers. Look at Batman, Spiderman, Superman and Catwoman: you wouldn't catch these omnipotent creatures baring vast expanses of flesh. They have got a tough job to do, and they need to be protected while at the same time looking sleek, invincible and mean!

Wearing black has always signified cruelty, wickedness or outlaw status. It's the colour of death, the opposite of purity. In Westerns, the bad guy always rides into town wearing a black hat. If you put your antihero in a black leather garment, he is immediately signified as being good in a scrap, perhaps a loner or outsider. In the film *The Wild One* Marlon Brando wears a black leather jacket, gets on his motorbike and gives birth to a fashion icon that has endured.

Wearing black leather has come to signify being bad. We know that the baddest bunch of all – the men who took black leather into another realm of taboo – was the SS. Always immaculate in their dress, uniforms spotless and polished and commanding absolute respect, the Nazis were the original power dressers. It cannot be ignored or denied that the uniform fetish of this most unpleasant group of fanatics lingers on and holds a fascination for people whose politics may well be democratic. These days, for obvious reasons, most fetish parties ban the wearing of Nazi chic. However, all the people I've spoken to who have expressed a liking for this look were keen to point out that they are tolerant, liberal individuals who have no desire to see fascism made reality; they merely like the cut of the cloth.

This regalia exudes a sexual appeal that maintains

the high sales of illustrated hardback coffee-table books of Nazi uniforms, Nazi regalia and the art of the third Reich, decades after its defeat. What part of our sexual psyches does this fascination tap into? Susan Sontag's analysis of 1972 still holds up: 'The SS was designed as an elite military community that would not only be supremely violent, but supremely beautiful.'[1] An arresting combination and one that has found its way into the iconography of much male gay sexual adventurism, from Genet's novel *Funeral Rites* through to the set dressing of leather bars of San Francisco. It is a powerful aesthetic. 'The colour is black, the material is leather, the seduction is beauty, the justification is honesty, the aim is ecstasy, the fantasy is death,' continues Sontag.[2]

Women, we have been conditioned to believe, are naturally disposed towards silk, satin and lace; the 'feminine' fabrics – flimsy garments that barely cover our sensitive bodies and show them off to best advantage. The subliminal message is that women – vulnerable, soft little things – aren't really tough at all. One material that has a controversial history is fur. Originally worn by both sexes to keep us warm during palaeolithic times, civilisation made us aware of the cruelty involved in procuring it, and since Sacher-Masoch dressed Wanda in animal pelts in *Venus in Furs*, fur acquired connotations of taboo, of being associated with cruel women and causing suffering. If we look at the paintings of the symbolist period of the late nineteenth century, particularly those of Gustave Moreau or Fernand Khnopff, there is usually some fur draped around the territory where frightening, all-powerful female subjects reign supreme. It would be unwise to upset one of Moreau's women; she would have your head on a plate if you scorned her.

In Khnopff's painting *The Caress*, the fur is the woman's own. She is a hybrid creature with the body of a leopard and the head of a woman. Her expression is one of sexual rapture. Frederick Sandys, an artist on the periphery of the Pre-Raphaelite circle, painted the famous Morgan le Fay, who sports a leopardskin around her waist as she uses her magical powers to unleash evil on her brother, King Arthur. Again, fur is associated with bad girls. Girls who are part animal, part predator. Fast forward to the 1950s and leopardskin becomes the trimming for any aspiring beat girl on the pull. It sends out a sexual message: 'I'm catlike and on the prowl. If you mess with me I'll hurt you; if you treat me right, you'll be rewarded with wild stuff.' Thankfully, most women are happy to wear fake fur these days. We can experiment with our wild side without having to harm endangered and beautiful creatures.

Some of the appeal of fetish fashion for women must be that it is empowering. You can feel pretty formidable in an all-in-one catsuit and boots in a way that is impossible if you are wearing a floaty dress and sandals. How much more threatening is the woman in black, shiny impenetrable hide than the easily torn feminine fabrics such as silk and satin. Leather and rubber are associated with toughness; of being a rebel or outsider or, specifically, a dominatrix. From Emma Peel in the British 1960s series *The Avengers* through to the industrial cyberfashion of late 1990s, an important factor in much female fetish clothing is the absence of vulnerability. This found its exhaltation in the late 1970s, when punk – the 'style in revolt' – incorporated accessories such as dog leads, chains, bondage loops on trousers, more zips than was necessary and materials such as plastic, lurex and, once more, fake fur.

The punkette was a bad girl; she wore her PVC

miniskirt too far up her thighs, her tights or stockings were ripped, and her make-up was theatrical, sometimes bordering on the grotesque. She was a pantomime parody of beauty; she wasn't putting herself on display to be fancied or adored by men. She wanted the antithesis to that standard response: to shock; to repel the male gaze; to deflect it. She didn't need a 'nice' boyfriend to justify her existence; she was quite happy making a noise on her own. For the first time in youth culture, aggressive clothing became the accepted dress code for girls as well as boys. It was fashion as anti-fashion, and it was an explosion of individuality. As Dick Hebdidge notes in his book *Subculture, The Meaning of Style*, '[punk rock fashion took] the illicit iconography of sexual fetishism ... from the boudoir, closet and pornographic film and placed on the street.'[3] Punk women adopted these trappings (stiletto heels, fishnet stockings, rubber capes and wet-look vinyl) and subverted their meaning. What was traditionally seen as enslaving became ripe for reappropriation and reinvention. That most illicit icon of all, the swastika, was purloined from the archives of bad taste and displayed as a symbol of rebellion. Not because punks were neofascist (in fact, the reverse was true, and the British Anti-Nazi League grew out of the embers of the punk movement) but because it showed that the youth were not afraid of nihilism. It could handle concepts of death and destruction and was prepared to tackle taboos head-on. Rather than hide from fear, punks gave it a face and a name. Vivienne Westwood and Malcolm McClaren called their fashion store Sex and sold heavy bondage gear, masks, chains, tit clamps and medical paraphernalia.

Twenty years on, women who wear rubber still raise eyebrows. When supermodel Naomi Campbell wore a rubber dress and high heels she was asked whether she thought such clothes were demeaning to women.

She quite rightly replied that, 'Grown women can do whatever they please.' I'll add to that, 'As long as it doesn't hurt anyone else or involve killing animals for their fur.'

Alison, 22, Student/Dancer

I fantasise at least once a day. I like to play with the image of a shy, virginal type who is taken by a bisexual guy who knows how to please her from A–Z. As far as I can remember, I have been turned on by shiny materials: nylon, leather and rubber, etc. I probably saw this on TV when I was quite young, before it was more common. I got into buying porn magazines and also enjoyed men in uniform and submissive men. I even put an advertisement in a paper to write to men who had motorbikes, as that was linked to my leather fetish.

My favourite fantasy goes like this. I've met this guy at a party. I go back to his place. We are both getting very hot and want each other. I take a shower and get into his bed; he disappears for five minutes and I start to wonder if he can read my mind. I'm falling asleep, only to turn around and find him dressed head to foot in shining black leather. Mmm! He has on a mask with eyeholes and a zipped mouth, gloves, a polo-necked short-sleeved top, leather trousers and black boots. By this time, I'm very wet and turned on. The smell and shininess is making me very horny. He takes my hand, starts stroking me and asks me if I like his leather fetish. He says that he thinks I'm the kind of woman who can handle this sex fetish. I answer yes, and then he asks me what I would like him to do. I reply that he can start by getting into bed with me. He does, feeling me all over with his strong body. I'm pretty turned on by the smell, the feel and the smoothness of his sexy outfit.

He goes down on me and I go down on him as he is

sitting on the edge of the bed. I get down on my hands and knees and suck him off, drinking in the smell of leather as he forces my head down. I suck him, feeling his thighs trembling as I give him pure pleasure. Afterwards, he spunks over my chest and I stand up and force him to lick every bit off my tits. Then I make him get on to all fours and I zip up his mask. I start to whip him until he puts up his hand to make me stop. Hearing his muffled screams has turned me on and made me very wet. He licks me out, pushing his tongue into me, and we have sex. He fucks me on top, then doggy-style, while rubbing my clit with his gloved hand. I then sit on his face, pressing and rubbing myself into his leather face and open mouth.

Belinda, 25, Unemployed
I tend to have recurring fantasies but they are usually about making love to my boyfriend. I used to get very turned on by men in uniform and would make love in very public places. These days I find biker types and long-haired 'arty' types particularly arousing. My current favourite fantasy is to meet my boyfriend from work and go home together. When we get in, we kiss tenderly and passionately. We have a bath together and make love in the bath. We then get dressed and go into the country on his bike. (He is dressed all in leather!) Once we are in a quiet spot, we slowly kiss, then make love over his bike.

Bridget, 25, Deputy Manager
I find tall leather-clad bikers and Goths very sexy, especially those with long hair and guitars. I also find uniforms a turn-on. A recurring fantasy of mine involves sex with my boyfriend and his three best mates. The story goes like this: All four guys stand naked in front of me, with their guitars in front of their dicks. I am blindfolded and have to tell one from the

other by sucking each one off. I would then like sex with them all at once!

Sharelle, 22, Homemaker
My fantasies tend to be all very different. My biggest turn-on, however, is leather, rubber and PVC. It has now become a fetish. I also find bikers extremely erotic. I had a very erotic experience once, when I was caught fucking on a motorbike by a group of hikers. We just carried on, the result being a group of gobsmacked hikers! My husband, after he has done his weight training, is gorgeous. He's all sweaty and smelly. I also find Madonna a tremendous turn-on. If she offered herself to me, I'd snap her up faster than ripping off my knickers.

I am a biker, as is my husband. My fantasy is to go to a bike rally kitted out in leather crotchless knickers, leather bustier with nipple cages, leather jeans and jacket. Once there, I enter into the wet T-shirt competition. I am stripped down to my crotchless studded leather thong. When my husband sees me, he gets rampantly horny and decides to take me on stage, on all fours, in front of forty to fifty thousand people. The music of Motorhead is belting out behind us. It is just myself and my husband, doing our own stage show in front of thousands. Then, a bloke asks if my husband wouldn't mind. Suddenly, there is a line of thousands queuing up to take me, or even just suck on my love juice. I get gang-banged for four days and three nights. When I get home, it's with a great big, shiny white smile on my face. My fantasy is at last fulfilled.

Kelly, 29, Midday Assistant
My husband and his friends come home from a night out and they all make love to me together. This is one of my recurring fantasies. Big bikes are a turn-on for me. I am dressed in black leather. The feel of the engine

vibrating between my legs, and the smell of leather filling my head, makes me wet.

Mary, 36, Administrative Assistant
I enjoy fantasies of being dominated, light bondage practises and discipline. It is important that I am, however, in control. Body piercing and anal sex also turn me on. Clothing is a major erotic influence. I like to see, feel and wear rubber, leather and vinyl, particularly as day-time fashion and not necessarily outrageous SM stuff.

The following is my story. It is a true story, although I have not used real names.

I met Lorraine at boarding school. We had both grown up on farms in northern Queensland. Farms there are very big, and the nearest neighbour is often a hundred or more kilometres away. High-school education was in the nearest town or city, and you had to be a boarder. I found myself sharing with Lorraine. At first we were homesick but soon took a liking to each other and became friends. We made it a habit to share a bed to comfort each other. It didn't take long to discover that pleasuring each other was far more exciting and satisfying than the solo exercises we were used to.

It wasn't until the second term that we discovered each other's secret sexual pleasures and imaginations. When at home on the farm, I discovered at an early age how calves were produced and I had witnessed the stallion cover the mares, and watched puppies and kittens being born. I soon found out how to pleasure myself, and took every possible opportunity to do so. I was also quite familiar with animals being chained: bulls having a ring put through their noses and horses being hobbled. These things started to play a role in my fantasies when masturbating. When I found a length of chain, I took it into my room and into bed. I imagined that I was being chained and punished while absolutely helpless. The chain became an important aid to mind-blowing orgasms. Returning to boarding school after the holidays, I took the chain with me. Lorraine found it when unpacking my suitcase.

I found that Lorraine had also packed some extras: a short leather belt, more like a paddle, and a riding crop. Lorraine had lost both her parents in a car accident and was living with her aunt and uncle. One time, waking up at night, she decided to go downstairs. Passing her aunt and uncle's bedroom she noticed a light shining through the door, which was slightly ajar. She also heard noises, which at first she didn't recognise. She couldn't resist the temptation to peep through the opening. Her aunt was receiving a good spanking from her husband. The moans she heard seemed to be expressing pleasure rather than pain. To her surprise, her aunt seemed to be making no effort to escape the punishment. When the spanking stopped, her uncle proceeded to caress her aunt in ways she knew, from her own exercises, could be very pleasant indeed. Her aunt, now on her hands and knees, was mounted by her uncle from behind. At this point her aunt looked up and saw her standing at the door. Before her aunt could react, Lorraine fled to her room, not knowing what to do, greatly embarrassed and mortified about what her aunt would do. At the same time, she was excited about what she had seen, and fantasised about how it would feel if she was subjected to this type of discipline.

She was to find out! Before she fell asleep again, her aunt came in, explaining as best she could what Lorraine had seen, telling her that she had been very naughty and would be punished the next day. And she was. Gradually, she made sure that she was regularly and sufficiently disobedient enough to be punished and experience the subsequent pleasure and intense orgasm that followed. Her aunt, though, never told her husband and, if she did, he never gave a sign that he knew.

Our mutual confessions were an excellent precursor for a very tiring night experimenting with our new-found toys. It was a good thing that classes did not start until two days later. We came to a decision; one week Lorraine would be the mistress and I would be her slave, the next week we would reverse the roles. After a satisfying session, Lorraine would need all her imaginative powers to explain why she couldn't join the swimming classes. I had, at times, similar problems when the chains left vivid marks.

[Some years later, Mary meets up again with Lorraine, who is now married.] We found that we were the same friends as before and that very little, if anything, had changed.

The arrangement between Lorraine and Charles was ideal. There was no doubt that Charles was the master and Lorraine his little slave. The pair also fitted out one of their rooms as a punishment room. Whenever we could, Lorraine and I continued our old games, but now with more sophistication, including dressing for pleasure. Charles had no objection, but it was a good way to punish Lorraine and make her extra happy. When Charles found me chained up in the punishment room, where Lorraine had left me on purpose, Lorraine and I both ended up with sore bottoms. Alas, it was only Lorraine who profited sexually from his treatment. I soon, however, added some excitement to these games by introducing both to my rubber and vinyl wardrobe [which Mary had bought while living in the UK].

I went out with a few guys, nice enough, but not what I wanted and needed; until the arrival of Alan, a friend of the pair, who was invited as a long-term houseguest. We got on all right but, although I was attracted to him, nothing happened. I thought it was time to test the waters. While up late talking and drinking wine, I spilled some red wine on Alan's shirt. This carelessness, Alan said, had to be punished and I was taken to the punishment room, chained and had my bottom attended to. (I suspected Lorraine had told on me.) As a consequence, we spent the night together and things developed. [Mary finds that Alan shares her love of dressing in rubber and vinyl and is well and truly hooked.]

We bought a house, got married and indulged in our rubber pastime whenever we could. The wedding took place at Charles and Lorraine's place. It was a simple affair with a few friends. What I did not realise was that there would be another ceremony of much greater importance to me. I was taken by Lorraine and her friend Marcia to change from my wedding outfit into something altogether different. They had selected a rather revealing outfit to wear to the coming ceremony. I put on my black bra with peep holes, panties with an open crotch, and my red dress, all in shiny latex. Over this, Marcia insisted I wore the black latex cape from my wardrobe. Marcia belonged to Dr Hedda. She assisted Dr Hedda as surgery assistant and was also her personal slave girl. When I was fully dressed, I was taken to the lounge room where a number of people had gathered, all belonging to a select circle of masters, mistresses and slaves. As I would learn, slaves could be borrowed, hired or auctioned. A friend of Alan's performed the ceremony. I was made to kneel before Alan and asked if I accepted him as my master. I agreed and was given a collar and whip to hand over to Alan as a token of my acceptance. Alan agreed to take me as his slave by placing the collar round my neck and hitting me seven times with the whip. Marcia had removed my cape and it was great to see Alan's look of surprise when he discovered my latex outfit – the one I had worn on our first rubber night. Since then, I have always been allowed to dress in latex, rubber, vinyl or leather when the mood grabs me.

I was told what was expected of me, and I was forced to pleasure each and every member of the circle. The next day we started our honeymoon, which confirmed my new status. We went to Dr Hedda's clinic and Alan said he wanted me to be pierced. When asked if I would consent, I replied that it was not up to me to give consent; I had to obey his wishes as commands. I could have refused, although that would mean I would no longer be a member of the circle, although our marriage would still be valid. Having met and married someone who at last met my needs, I agreed to wear the rings he had selected. There would be seven: one through each nipple and two at the top of my vagina through the outside lips. These last two were mainly decorative. Heavier ones were to be inserted in my inside lips. They could be used to tie me up or to hold a padlock, whatever my master had in mind. A smaller one would go through my clitoris. It made me think of the cattle at home, and I asked Alan if, as a favour, I could have a ring through my nose. A hole was made in the septum, which would allow a ring to be inserted any time Alan considered it necessary.

Under the skilled expertise of Dr Hedda and the loving care of Marcia, the pain was not too bad. The first few days, I was not to serve Alan. After that he could use my mouth for a week, then my bottom was available for about a week, as well. If the wounds had healed satisfactorily, after about another week he would have complete use of me. Returning home, I found Lorraine had organised a party for the circle, where I was to show my piercings, and a start was made with slave training. I also found that I had a new job as a legal secretary, for which I was qualified. I would be employed by Alex, a Queen's counsel. He would have full use of me but could not punish me. I would have to keep track of any and all errors I made. This would be compared to Alex's record. If both were the same Alan would punish me at home accordingly. If there were discrepancies the punishment would be doubled. Unlike Lorraine, who had some choice, I had to wear a collar of some sort or other at all times. Also, I had to wear latex or vinyl whenever possible, wear no panties, and, if I did, they should be crotchless.

Alex's wife was also in the circle and submissive to Alan. However, she could – and did – lord it over me. She certainly knew how to excite me with a riding crop or paddle. It is now Sunday afternoon. We slept in after a late dinner and exhausting circle activities. I am sitting at the computer, writing these notes in my favourite blue latex kaftan. Around my waist is a chain with another chain going between my legs and up between my bottom cheeks to join against the waist chain. Last night I was well used and, as a result, my sex and bottom were slack and open. Alan wanted me to stay like that and has inserted a dildo in both apertures, held in place by the chain. Alan has just ordered me to get him a drink. In the meantime, he has read my notes and found mistakes and errors which, he says, show my carelessness. Correction, he says, is called for. I have knelt in front of him and he has inserted the nose ring. It raises my expectation and excitement, and the inside of my kaftan is getting wet. I can certainly expect a sore bottom. This is the end of my story.

Caroline, 37, Unemployed

When I was about fourteen I developed an obsession with Nazi uniforms, although it had nothing to do with being racist; I wasn't. I longed to be stripped and interrogated by good-looking Nazi officers and would make sure that I saw every World War II film and the series *Manhunt* on TV. I would imagine that the Nazis would initiate me into their secret inner circle and we would fuck brutally day and night. All the trappings of German fascism aroused me: from the sleek black Mercedes cars to the death's head insignia on the peaked caps. I also loved the idea of pure German girls, with their hair in plaits and wearing dark, sober school uniforms, having lesbian sex with me. I took to learning German as a teenager and began to buy Nazi medals and regalia from antique shops. This freaked my parents out something rotten, and no one could understand my fascination apart from a friend's older sister, who admitted she was interested in Nazis. She was into heavy metal and helped me to lose my virginity. I've seen the terrible footage of what happened in the concentration camps and there's no way anyone can defend their politics. The reality of fascism is evil. However, why is it that a swastika armband can get me aroused even now? I once had a sexual relationship with a Jewish man, and he was into SM. When he confessed that Nazis were his fantasy, too (he was bisexual), I felt better about my own fantasies. It has to be the ultimate taboo. And I guess that is why I like it. When I saw the film *The Night Porter* I felt my fantasy was not as uncommon as I'd been led to believe.

These days any smart uniform is a turn-on for me, except for British police with their bobby helmets, which are just ridiculous. I like US traffic cops, which is quite a common fantasy. I think my fantasies tend to be more like gay men's fantasies. I like the image of construction workers, cops, boot boys and military men. In real life, however, I wouldn't want to give them the time of day. It's a funny thing, sexuality, isn't it?

Jacqueline, 39, Teacher

I find imagining that I have an audience a real turn-on. It is usually, but not always, my boyfriend. He talks me through my masturbation, instructing and watching. I love sexy underwear: stockings and suspenders, but not crotchless panties. I also love leather clothing but not leather underwear. My only male-assisted method of achieving orgasm is oral sex received from my boyfriend. I get off on images of penetration and erections and particularly images of people performing oral sex. There is also something very erotic about illicit sex and the fear of discovery, along with the anticipation of sex and the moment of penetration. When I was younger, I found Yul Bryner very erotic, and I still get hot flushes when I think of him now.

The following is not so much a fantasy as something I wish to do. I want to tie up my boyfriend – who is a distinguished, grey-haired businessman – using his silk ties. One of the ties should be around his neck, one used to blindfold him. He may be sitting or lying down. I then smear his penis with toffee-flavoured ice cream and fellate him. After this he must give me oral sex while still blindfolded. I am smeared with the ice cream. My boyfriend needs to be blindfolded because I want him to concentrate on touch rather than sight. Ideally, the whole act should take place in front of a large mirror. Throughout I am very dominant and am wearing a basque and stockings, etc. In reality my boyfriend isn't the dominating type, and I have to try to make him dominate me. I want to be commanded and forced to do things.

'Miss P', 22, Personnel Administrator

I like fantasising about women's submission to men, especially well-muscled men in uniforms. Involved in these fantasies are images of arousal and foreplay, heightening the anticipation of penetration. Restriction and spanking are recurring scenarios. My current favourite fantasy includes all these combinations: a rich guy employs girls to look after his house. All the girls wear maids' outfits and stockings and suspenders without knickers. He comes back from work to find one girl dusting the furniture; he talks to her while feeling her up. She then gives him a blow job while another girl is instructed to lick the first girl's clit.

When he's ready, he bends the first girl over the coffee table, slaps her arse and proceeds to take her from behind, pumping into her until he comes. He then turns her over; she is lying on the coffee table, her knees spread. He kneels between her legs. He uses a candle as a dildo and proceeds to flick her clit until she comes, too. The other girl gets nasty because she hasn't been serviced, so he takes her upstairs, lays her down and uses jelly to insert love balls inside her. He arouses her and then leaves her. The next day he gets in from work and calls this girl into the study. He makes her rock backward and forward, causing her to become aroused and her juices to flow. He then strips her, blindfolds her and invites two of his workmates into the room. He lays her down, takes out the love balls and allows a threesome to take place while he watches. Both guys screw her on top and from behind. She rides them and takes them in her mouth. All the time there are hands and mouths everywhere.

Vampires, Beasts and Other Beings

'Sex reeking with the full perfume of the swamp . . .'
Prof. Leonard Wolf (*The Annotated Dracula*,
New York, 1975)

Vampire fantasies are a hardy perennial of the sexual imagination. From the British Hammer Horror films of the early 70s, which played out every interpretation of Bram Stoker's *Dracula*, through to Tom Cruise bringing

Anne Rice's Lestat to life in *Interview With a Vampire*, the virile undead lover has entranced many generations of women. One cannot forget Catherine Deneuve and Susan Sarandon's vampiric lesbian affair in *The Hunger* – surely one of most erotic films ever made. The early Hammer films were heavy on sexual symbolism, rather than being explicit. The vision of Christopher Lee sinking his fangs into Caroline Munro's lovely neck in *Dracula AD 1972* was many adolescents' first turn-on. Vampires are the ultimate existential antiheroes. There is a poignancy to their fragile existence. They hold the secret of everlasting life but they are constantly beset by sadness, living a twilight existence and trapped into an unending routine of having to slake their hunger.

The vampire is undeniably and powerfully attractive. This mythical creature gave its name to the seductive woman; the vamp. Whether male or female, they are always so potent; always in a state of animal arousal. We desire them, we empathise with their vulnerability and usually feel sad rather than relieved when Dr Van Helsing or a similar 'good guy' drives the stake through their hearts; when the forces of Christian goodness banish these dark lords and deadly femmes fatales of the underworld. A number of Hollywood movies, such as *The Lost Boys* and *Near Dark*, have taken the vampire out of the Gothic castle and placed him in suburban America, thereby giving a new lease of life to what was seen as a European fable. The idea that the all-American boy can be as vulnerable to the vampire's kiss as the swooning Victorian lady makes room for a whole new creed of vampire lovers.

It did not surprise me that women sent in fantasies based on the vampire story. In some cases the subjects told me they went some way to making the fantasy real. Elena confessed to dressing in black mourning clothes and making love in cemeteries late at night in the hope of having a supernatural sexual experience.

Franklin D Roosevelt once said, 'The only thing to fear is fear itself.' When we are very young, it's natural to fear death and the ghoulish inhabitants of our nightmares. The unknown can hold all manner of frightening evils. As adults, however, we can learn to stare terror in the face and make palatable characters out of scary monsters and the terrifying undead; to transform them into products for our amusement and entertainment. One way of doing this is by eroticising the fearful. Many of the physiological reactions of being scared are the same as those which occur when we are sexually aroused: perspiration; a rapid heart-beat; a dry mouth; dilated pupils etc., so it's understandable why some people choose to mix a little fear into their fantasies for an extra *frisson*. This is not the only reason, of course, but it's true to say that products such as suspense and horror films have a definite and lurid sexual appeal. One only has to watch the films of Mario Bava, Dario Argento or David Cronenberg to realise this.

Our relationship with fear is a complex part of the human psyche. On the one hand we recoil from it while at the same time we actively desire to 'know the worst' – looking through our fingers as we cover our eyes during the scary bits in horror films. We don't want to admit that we often get a thrill from being scared. Human curiosity has its own ghoulish side, and it would be a naive person who declared that no one wants to hear the 'juicy bits' of a story.

Moing on to another taboo, the commonly held idea that bestial fantasies are about rolling around in mud with pigs and goats is a mile short of the mark. The few women who sent in fantasies involving animals are influenced more by fairy tales and anthropological knowledge of practices such as shamanism than sleazy 1970s colour super8 movies filmed on the farm.

Take, for instance, Gina's fantasy about coupling with a puma and giving birth to a creature, half puma, half girl, who becomes an environmental vigilante. This is a new kind of fantasy that identifies Gina more as an eco-warrior than as a pervert. The dominant notion in the section is that the non-human partner is some kind of ideal. The creature is in some way superior to mere mortals and absolutely preferable to the human male.

Madeline, 21, Barmaid

Mostly I think about making love to a woman and also having brutal sex with a vampire who has just bitten me. My first turn-ons were sexy vampire films. I like having sex to the music of Aerosmith. I wish I could be more open and not think it's dirty to have these thoughts. I would like to meet a man who would laugh and share my fantasy. It would be really good if I could have an orgasm. I don't think I've ever had one and I'm sure I never will.

In my fantasy I am lying in bed and, just as I'm going to sleep, something is moving up my body. I open my eyes and it's a lovely, sexy, long-haired man. He's a vampire with red eyes, and he kisses me and then he bites my neck. When we have sex, it is so good. Then I slowly turn into a vampire myself and we carry on having sex.

Marie, 34, Community Care Support Assistant

A recurring theme in my fantasies is of male homosexual intercourse, but only without my involvement. I also find men shaving very arousing, as I do spontaneous occasions; for example, being taken unawares in non-sexual circumstances. I sometimes still get off on certain films and actors, such as Al Pacino in *Sea of Love* and Marlon Brando in *Last Tango in Paris*. I remember also being turned on by watching lovers in Rome. A theme that is apparent in my current favourite fantasy is unfulfilled desire. This current fantasy is based on Louis, the vampire in *Interview With a Vampire*. It is very much the character of Louis and not the actor, Brad Pitt, who turns me on. I fell in love/lust with him before Hollywood made the film.

In my fantasy the vampire's face is hazy, but I know his character is Louis'. It's almost as if I want to be Lestat, to feel close to him. Louis loves me, but he cannot drink my blood. I'm his woman. My fantasy is more about what doesn't happen. I beg, plead and throw myself at Louis, but he loves me too much to hurt me. He doesn't want to destroy me and condemn me to his hated existence. Penetration will do this; it will turn me into one of the undead. As far as Louis is concerned, he can't let it happen. We can touch, caress, kiss and even perform oral sex, but the sheer frustration of not being penetrated is immense, so we spend hours compensating. For some reason – a psychologist would love this – I find unfulfilled sex a big turn-on. In the fantasy, even though we can't have each other, we can find release with alternative partners: me with a faceless dick and him anally with Lestat. Fulfilment is, however, only delayed and my reaction is to end with forcing Louis to take me completely – and so we become one for eternity.

Elena, 29, Bank Clerk
It is dusk. I wake up on a cold steel table in a cold white room unsure of my whereabouts and unable to speak. My entire body aches. I realise that I'm strapped down. In the room are large jars filled with golden liquid and a smaller steel trolley covered with bizarre-looking instruments. I lie there in confusion for about an hour. I squint around this dimly lit room and see the word 'embalming fluid' written on one of the

bottles. I panic. I am writhing and gasping to make a noise.

Two tall thin young men enter the room. They are dressed in full Victorian undertakers' dress: long black coats, cravats, and top hats with black sashes tied around them. One is wearing tiny blacked-out spectacles. They tell me that everyone thinks that I'm dead and that they are going to keep it that way. I am dressed entirely in black mourning dress; my hair is in an upsweep with black and white satin roses. My skin looks deathly pale. They tell me that they have weighted my coffin down with bricks and that they will be conducting a horse-drawn funeral for me tomorrow.

One of the men begins to touch me and feel the line of my breasts through my tight dress. The other runs his hand along my leg, forcing my skirts up over my stomach. The man with the dark glasses moves his face close to mine and begins to unhook my dress from the front. My dress is then cut from my body. My breasts are roughly grabbed and pulled up from beneath my whalebone corset. I am fed with opium and absinthe. They say very little but I know they are going to keep me and use me as their plaything. I will live in the cellars beneath the funeral parlour. In a semi-conscious daze I can feel them both begin to go to work on me with grasping hands and thrusting fingers.

Anon, 25, Library Assistant
I used to be turned on by a schoolteacher who had sexy, tight trousers and a big bulge. String vest tops that reveal the skin underneath are sexy. Some Mills & Boon books are a riveting read. Other turn-ons include voyeurism, animals shagging in a field, people showing affection in public and any films with a sex scene. Today voyeurism is still a feature of my fantasies; I particularly get turned on by the idea of sex or foreplay

in public places and punk rocker dress. The latter must be related to a bondage fetish.

Here is my favourite fantasy. The sun is shining and I'm lying on the beach. My body is getting warm from the heat. I get up and gracefully enter the water, allowing it to cool me down. I look around and, seeing I am alone, I throw away my bikini. The feel of the water flowing around my body is lovely. I lie on my back and allow myself to relax. Without realising, I feel my own fingers inside me and I begin to get excited. Suddenly, I feel something brush against my leg. I raise my head and feel something run up inside my thigh. I feel its slippery, rough tongue begin to lick at my femaleness. I look up and realise that Flipper the dolphin has come back to me. He must have sensed my womanly smell in the water.

He is as excited as me and, without warning, the large mammal enters me. He is so large that at first I think I'm going to burst. Within seconds I can feel him flowing inside me. He pulls out and swims off, nodding his head in the distance. I lie there, near the peak of my desire, knowing he will return with his friends.

Jennifer, 25, Student
I love the idea of being a mermaid and luring men to my undersea kingdom. I've thought about making love with a dolphin. I've seen films of these marvellous creatures sporting erections. They are very intelligent and would make sensitive lovers. I would rather have sex with a dolphin that the average man one finds in a provincial nightclub on a Saturday evening. As far as brains go, there is no competition.

I would love to be able to swim underwater indefinitely, coupling as if in an aquatic ballet with a young male dolphin. I've heard that their penises are rough and serrated, so maybe it wouldn't be as comfortable as I'd like. I like the visual images conjured up by the mythology of the sea: the sirens, leviathans, Atlantis and marine-boy, etc. When I was a little girl I would daydream about finding an undersea kingdom and being made a princess so I would never have to go back to school. I would be made into a mermaid and would spend all day swimming and decorating myself with jewels and treasures of the deep. As I grew up these fantasies became sexualised and began to include elements of capture and imprisonment: me capturing sailors from shipwrecks and dragging them deep into my lair, where they would be made to pleasure me and my mermaid friends all day, every day, until they died of exhaustion or escaped. There was a TV ad recently for Levis jeans that featured this scenario. It must be part of a collective unconscious of female fantasy.

Gina, 32, Office Worker

I'm fascinated by the idea of inter-species sex. Not the unpleasant, unhygienic farmyard stuff, but the genuinely beautiful idea of coupling with a wild beast, such as a big cat. I saw a television programme once that featured a couple of leopards at it, and it blew my mind. They seemed to be enjoying it totally; the female was howling and purring and pawing her mate, who was pumping his furry hindquarters like a jackhammer! He was gorgeous and, when he came, there was a look of total rapture on his face. I would love to mate with a furry creature. I visited Prague zoo and stared for ages at the tigers. They had lovely furry balls, apricot coloured and heavy, and it was as much as I could do to prevent myself from crawling into the pen and giving them a rub.

In my animal fantasy, I am with a puma or leopard. I am camping in a remote area and, when night falls, a beautiful beast comes to me. Although I am human, he doesn't attack me because I can communicate with him. I can tap directly into his soul, like a sexual shaman. I let him chase me, tackle me to the ground and fuck me. I can feel the heat, strength and warmth of that furry body. He bites me, but not too savagely, and climaxes spectacularly. I imagine what it would be like to give birth to a special cat-like she creature – much more attractive than a human baby – that I would then release into the wild to be brought up by the big cats as a lithe sexy puma girl. She would terrorise men who destroy sacred lands and kill our beautiful wild animals. She would lure them with her good looks then mate with them before savagely ripping them to shreds and eating them.

Ally, 49, Massage Therapist
I am bisexual and I would say that I am semi-aroused (or so it seems) most of the time. I like masterful, sexually dominating men and strong, attractive, clever, middle-aged women. I first discovered my sexual nature at eight or nine years old. I remember enjoying a black and white film in which a Native American was tough on a female, throwing away her moccasins so she couldn't follow him. He eventually relented and showed her tenderness later. Pain turning to pleasure is a constant theme in my fantasies; harsh words replaced with tenderness and loving afterwards. S&M features widely, as do stories of schoolgirls being caned by lesbian mistresses.

The title of my favourite fantasy of the moment is 'Space Whore' and I'm one of the best! I live in the future, where certain girls are trained to be space whores. They are chosen because of their suitability: being highly sexed, love juices always flowing, etc. They have to be intelligent enough to study psychology to degree level. They are assigned to spaceships and crews who need them for relief. Their role is to accommodate both male and female crew members, so they have to be genuinely bisexual. Space whore is not a derogatory term in the future. She is a highly intelligent sex therapist and facilitator. Imagine the sheer pleasure!

Darlene, 32, Housekeeper/Nanny

My recurring fantasy is of sex with a hermaphrodite. I get the best of both worlds. When I was thirteen, I saw the movie *Star Wars*. For the next six months, all I could think about was Darth Vader and I having sex. I never quite got over it. I always went for the bad guys. Some of my favourite turn-ons now are more basic. One of them is sex with a good-looking man or woman (or both) in a kilt in the highlands of Scotland.

My favourite fantasy takes place one night when I am taking a walk and I see a strange light in a clearing. I go a little closer for a look and suddenly start being pulled into the light. There is a doorway to another world. When I go through, I see ten men and two women waiting for me. They tell me that I am the first to come to their world. They take me to their king and queen. Along the way I have sex every three hours. It is a twelve-hour trip. When I finally meet the king and queen they tell me that I cannot go back home as the door only works one way. To ease the pain of homesickness, they give me the ten men and two women as my slaves and I live a horny and happy life.

Anna, 22, Export Administrator

When I was younger I didn't have particular fantasies, only scent and making love to someone I trusted. These days trust is still important. Laughter and sexy books are also turn-ons.

Let me tell you my favourite fantasy. I imagine a man and a woman, who are strangers, being kidnapped by a cult that keeps them apart but continuously taunts and flirts with them. In the meantime, they are strapped up and cannot touch themselves.

They are shown erotic films, books and pictures and are driven almost insane with lust. Finally they are strapped naked to boards and lowered into a pit. They are surrounded by the cult and can only touch body to body. Slowly, they are given permission to lick, kiss and then touch each other. They are then given toys, etc., before getting down to it. This leads to lots of orgies and gay/lesbian scenes. The couple then remains in the cult to live out its unleashed fantasies!

Total Taboo

Maddie, 52, Unemployed

I have a very definite recurring theme to my fantasies: incest. I am in the shower when my dad comes in for a pee, as is his usual way when I am showering. He stands facing me and I get out of the shower and dry myself. Usually, I go straight to bed and Dad goes back downstairs, but tonight he lightly knocks on my door. 'Let me feel your beautiful breasts,' he says.

'Not now,' I reply. 'Mother's downstairs. Wait till she goes to work tomorrow, then you can do what you like.'

'Let's have a quick feel,' he says and fondles me quickly. He asks me to open my legs, then he slides his hand in and quickly touches me. 'Pull up my kilt and touch my cock,' he pleads, and I give him a quick feel. He leaves after a moment but returns in half an hour, knocking on my door and saying, 'I've come to tell you about the phone call Mother's just had. Her friend is coming out of hospital and she is going to meet her; she's catching the train tonight. I'm driving her to the station in a moment.'

While he is talking, his hands are under the bedclothes, touching me between my legs. He gets a surprise as I have a vibrator inside me. He pulls it out and inserts his fingers instead, making me come and kissing me to stop me crying out. He licks his fingers and enjoys the taste of it. He asks me if, when he gets back, I will let him suck me off.

'Only if you promise to put this in me and make me come,' I reply, while rubbing his cock.

'I'd love to,' he says, 'but I dare not make you pregnant.'

'Don't worry, I need an operation before I can have a baby.' We both look forward to his return from the drive. I'm waiting in his bed for him when he gets home. He comes in quickly and undresses himself. I sit on the edge of the bed and take his beautiful cock in my mouth and suck it while squeezing his balls.

'Enough,' he says. 'I'll come if you carry on, and I want to be inside you so much.'

Naturally he doesn't last long and we both come together. We don't get much sleep that night as we do it every way we can. He takes me up the arse and comes in my mouth and between my large breasts (38E cup).

The next weekend we visit his two brothers, who live on a farm. One is divorced, one widowed. We all enjoy a great weekend of fucking and sucking, sometimes one to one, other times all together. I enjoy taking one in my cunt, one in my mouth and one up my arse at the same time. It is good when we all come together.

Jocelyn, 61, Retired

I'm very happy to be able to enjoy my very secret and previously undisclosed fantasies. I couldn't bear the shame of anyone finding out. Being an older woman, I was brought up to think of sex in any shape or form as unsavoury. I have always found anything to do with the male organ arousing. Men urinating, or becoming obsessed with their own and others' penises, has been recurringly arousing for me. I like to think about men taking great delight in their penises or being competitive about them: urinating, masturbating, seeing how far and how high they can pee and come, or men pissing on each other in combat, or on women during foreplay – and finding sadistic pleasure in this. I imagine a young streetwise girl instigating sex with four fishermen, then being joined by her voluptuous, sophisticated, sexy mother. The combinations are endless, and I imagine them having sex in various positions and being joined by the girl's father, who is extremely well endowed, knowledgeable and bisexual.

I also think about a guesthouse with children, parents and grandparents and they are all completely uninhibited. They all participate in realising their sexual desires, which include lesbianism, homosexuality and bisexuality. The house has a gardener who has an insatiable desire and has his penis out every half an hour, either peeing or masturbating or having sex with women, men, children and animals. He loves his penis and has a constant desire to put it through its paces as often as possible. He loves an audience.

I can pinpoint the origin of my fantasies to when I was at primary school. The toilets were outside and the boys' urinal was immediately in front of the girls' loos. There was no partition and so the girls could sit on the toilets and watch the boys peeing. The boys loved to show off, too, and have an audience with each other. Sometimes, some of them would pee on the girls and all the girls would scream in mock horror. This memory has stuck with me all my life.

Chapter Eight

Loving Ourselves to Bits: Exhibitionism and Being Adored

I am giddy, expectation whirls me round.
The imaginary relish is so sweet
That it enchants my sense.
    William Shakespeare, *Troilus and Cressida*,
                (1602) act 3, sc. 2

A large group of respondents sent in fantasies that are about being adored for showing off their sexual selves. These are the fantasies that are about having super-confidence or star quality; gaining hordes of admirers with the minimum of effort. In real life, we rarely get the chance to safely and blatantly show off our desirability in public; for a start, we would want to choose our audience. Most of us are hampered by shyness and the fear of rejection – not to say ridicule or scorn. Unrequited lust can weigh heavily on our egos, and a sober declaration of sexual attraction is a risky business in the mating game. We often need a little courage in the form of a drink or two before we can stutter out invitations for a coffee: the sub-text of which everyone knows but still pretends to take on face value.

Women are not conditioned into making the first move, although many men now tell us that they would prefer us to be more obvious in our seduction. For many women, the idea of admitting to being the sexual predator is galling. We might as well have a notice stamped our foreheads saying, 'I'm a filthy slut and I'm dying for it.' The paradox is that if men need sex, they need to seek it with a partner who is presumably 'lacking in virtue'. As Nancy Friday points out in *Women on Top*, 'To combine sex and familial love in one woman makes her too powerful, and him too little.'[1] Attitudes are changing for the better around this issue, I'm sure, although many men still fear the confident sexual woman. The thought of our object of desire refusing our advances is daunting for both sexes, although men are more likely to shrug off rejection better than women; they think, She's the one that's missing out, whereas we may blame ourselves for being undesirable in some way.

Men are encouraged from an early age to 'have a go' and 'get stuck in' while girls are kept back and warned not to make fools of themselves. There's part of us as women that isn't comfortable with being thought of as sexually demanding. We will joke with our girlfriends about being voracious, but we are wisely cautious when expressing our sexual selves to men. Many women know it is prudent to reveal their sexuality a little at a time. This may be our genetic memories working with our best interests at heart. It has long been thought that men need sex in a way that women don't; and those women who match or overtake the desire men see as their privilege have been vilified, lampooned and feared. We're also taught to create an air of mystery about ourselves; to not give away too much too soon, lest our conquest lose interest early on in the game. How many cartoons have we seen where the wily old coyote leaps through hoops and does backflips to impress the cool, calm and collected sex kitten who is idly buffing her nails or reading a magazine?

The irony is that she wants him as badly as he wants her, but no one's letting on. The command a woman can exercise over her admirers allows her to pick and choose. This is where women find their dominance; it is the power tool of female sexuality. We cannot resist having an effort made for our attentions. Although a large number of fantasies in this book appear to be about being sexually submissive, the overwhelming majority are also about being adored. The most popular female fantasy is to have control over a man through the fact that he desires you so desperately. While fundamentalist feminists and moralists rage about women being stripped of power by being portrayed as merely sexual, most women are smart enough to know the truth about how that power works, and that there are two categories of dominance: physical and psychic. While men enjoy the former, women wipe the board with the latter. We know that however powerful or politically correct men purport to be, they will respond to overt sexual signals. They simply cannot help themselves. A woman would rarely let down her guard or succumb to sexual desire in the way that heads of state, spies and military personnel have done over the centuries at the flimsiest promise of sexual favours. Most men think with their dicks and want their lusts instantly satisfied so they can move on. Woman's Achilles' heel is that she is vulnerable to flattery but she wants to bask in the glory for as long as possible; to be told that she looks nice, that he loves spending time with her, that he has eyes for her alone.

Successful seduction is about good timing. Women

tend to be patient, and cunning, more cat-like; not leaping too soon like some over-friendly hound with his tongue hanging out. We unconsciously check out the desirability of everyone who passes us on the street, categorising and selecting, filing and judging. Most men will openly admit to unconsciously rating every woman's desirability on a scale of one to ten. There is a popular game in 'new lad' culture called 'How many pints . . .?', the remainder of the question being '. . . would you have to drink before having sex with her?'

The way women form opinions of people's attractiveness is usually more furtive and subtle than the eye-boggling gawp of men. However, it's that eye-boggling gawp that the women in this section actively want to see in many of their fantasies. Some go as far as wanting to be the subject in sex-education lessons; being prodded and inspected before a spellbound audience of excited young men. These fantasies are about wanting to be worshipped; to be held up as an ideal of desirability. One could say it's an unfair society that rewards people for their attractiveness above all else, but those rewards are what many of us are rushing to attain. The cosmetics and dieting industries make billions out of our desire to be gorgeous, while at the same time playing on our insecurities about wrinkles, unwanted hair and excess pounds. We want sexual approval, and we are prepared to spend heavily to get it.

There's something very therapeutic about these fantasies in that they act as tools of self-affirmation for the women who have them. If we're constantly being presented with the ideal formula of how women should look, it's good to fantasise about being adored for who we are. Chloe's fantasy of performing on stage with a male stripper is marvellous. She gets a thunderous applause at the end of the show. They are enjoying themselves through her. Her role in the fantasy is the desire of all the women in the audience.

This culture of ideals – of acquisitiveness, perpetual youth, speed, fitness and wealth – can leave us feeling miserable about ourselves if we perceive that we're lacking in any of those areas. We have to be psychically strong to fight off the depression that is a natural result of living in a society where value judgements are based on shallow criteria. The high circulation of magazines featuring the lifestyles of the wealthy and famous means that we are continually fascinated by what the rich and beautiful are doing. I cannot imagine these privileged subjects purchasing the bottom-shelf week-lies aimed at the people the ad-men call C3s (the lower-income bracket), filled as they are with stories of trauma, disease and heartbreak.

Many of us give ourselves a hard time trying to realise unattainable goals in all areas of our lives. This is why our imaginations are important, and why it's good to fantasise about being adored, fancied and valued, whatever our age, body shape, sexuality, race or class. A bit more self-love – in the most holistic sense of the expression – is what we can all use more of.

Michaela, 35, Housewife/Mother
I like to fantasise about two or more men. They are restrained in some way, either physically or mentally, from touching me, until I allow it. I love wearing short skirts, preferably black leather, along with sheer tights, high-heeled boots or shoes. I get off on seeing men's reactions. Their age doesn't matter. When I realised my legs were my best asset, there was no stopping me. These days I can get turned on by anything out of the ordinary. Things I shouldn't be doing, people I shouldn't be seeing, anything apart from being a housewife and mum.

My favourite fantasy begins with me dancing in a nightclub. I am the only girl dancing. There are a group of blokes, all as horny as hell, watching. I dance towards them and pick one of them to dance with. We get very erotic and start to undress each other. Another bloke comes over. He is behind me and starts to put his hands on my breasts. The other kneels on the floor and takes my skirt off. I am only wearing stockings and suspenders and am still dancing very slowly and erotically.

By now the first bloke has removed my top and bra. All the other guys in the club are standing and watching. I realise I am extremely turned on and soaking wet. The bloke who is kneeling pulls me towards him and flicks his tongue between my legs, just licking the tops of my thighs. Then I push him down and sit on his face. The other guy is now kissing my breasts, throat and face. Suddenly I feel hands all over me, stroking and touching, taking off my stockings and sucking my toes. I seem to explode and come and come. All of these horny blokes want to eat my pussy. They think I'm the best thing on two legs. They all adore me.

Felicity, 32, Civil Servant
I like to fantasise several times a day and one of my recurring themes is meeting someone where the sexual attraction is so overwhelming that it transcends all other emotions. I used to get very aroused by all the precursors to a sexual encounter, or a possible one, such as putting on make-up and perfume, and feeling attractive and confident. It is also a real turn-on to be introduced to someone you find attractive and finding you have things in common. I love being made to feel special and attractive.

My husband makes me very aroused. I also like reading erotic love stories to my husband. My favourite fantasies involve being irresistible. Just the sight of an attractive, though not necessarily good-looking man, is generally enough to stir my imagination. My favourite recurring fantasy is to arrive at a meeting and be instantly attracted to someone else there. The feeling, of course, is mutual.

Teresa, 29, Housewife

I like to fantasise about having sex with my husband and another man at the same time. I enjoy reading porn and like getting off on nude male bodies, especially their dicks. Black Lace books are my favourites. My husband hates it because I can't keep off his dick when I read them. Any time, any place, anywhere. Just call me the Martini lady! I like sex with vibrators, and sex in open garages or fields. I get particularly turned on when a man has just got out of the bath and is nice and clean.

My favourite fantasy starts off by game playing. My man's been out drinking with my brother. He comes back to my house and climbs into bed beside me and begins to lick at my pussy. I begin to wake up and get slightly wet. I then return the favour at the same time. He then enters my anus, while messing with my G-spot. I play with myself at the same time. Afterwards, we have a good session with the vibrator and full-blown sex. He then goes back to using the vibrator on me while I take him in my mouth and start to lick, suck and give him a good gobble. The next thing, the bedroom door opens and in walks Mr Postman with nothing on his bottom half and a huge erection.

My God! I think, I'm in for the time of my life. He tells my partner to move over, and we start again. Only this time it's the real thing, instead of the vibrator, and I can't wait for the dustmen to call the day after. After them the window cleaners come to watch and then have a go to see if they can do any better. Let me at them all!

Kitty, 42, Manager

I tend to have some recurring themes in my fantasies. They include being very cleverly seduced by a man or a woman and very specific sexual clothing, such as lingerie, garters, miniskirts, and see-through or tight tops. I also like the idea of being on display or being a voyeur and, perhaps, in the process, learning something of sexual techniques. Another fantasy is of being a concubine in a harem, attempting to seduce the sultan. I would like to say that one of the things that endears me to Black Lace books is the warning about safe sex versus fantasy in the front of each book. As I'm sure you understand, fantasies are often just that. Some situations are not ones that women would like to find themselves in in real life. It's important for men to know that it is wrong to force a woman sexually, despite any fantasy she may have that uses such scenarios.

My favourite fantasy is somewhat vague. I am in some sort of very comfortable restraint, and lying on a couch, wearing Victorian clothes. I have been seduced into being here through very careful planning. No brutish strength is involved. Here I am and the decision has been made for me. There are two or three men in the room: a teacher in his 30s or 40s and one or two students in their early 20s. Naturally, they are all attractive or sexy, though not in the typical Hollywood sense. They are all wearing suits. Perhaps this is a training school for monks re-entering the world, or a very special kind of prep school. The older man is teaching the others how to be with a woman. I'm basically a visual aid. Sometimes in my fantasy the older man and I have had some kind of a relationship, and sometimes he has never met me before. He is not overly talkative, but his tone is quiet and patient.

The older man begins to undress me slowly, just a little. Occasionally he makes a comment to the students; perhaps about how he is kissing me, perhaps to remind them that kissing and nibbling should be gentle and light, in order to leave me wanting more. He slowly kisses my neck, barely breathes across my shoulder and gently nuzzles down a strap of the dress I'm wearing. He mouths my breast through the thin fabric of the dress and sucks on my nipple. He then nuzzles his head between my breasts and gently draws down the top of my dress. He is very slow, deliberate and tantalising, sometimes just breathing hot air across the erogenous zones around my breasts.

He carefully but firmly pulls up my dress from the bottom, touching the backs of my knees and slowly moving up my cream-coloured stockings to the very top, kissing my bare thigh. He quietly tells the others that all women are different, and that they must carefully pay attention to responses in order to determine which part of a woman's body is crying out for more. 'For example,' he says, 'you notice when I leave her breasts for her thighs, she will want me back to her breasts again, because you can see how they're reaching out.' (My nipples are feeling a bit abandoned and are, indeed, reaching out for the lost caress.)

He is not gentle so much as careful and deliberate. Once or twice the others ask if they can also feel, especially when he is putting his lips around my clitoris, tasting the different parts of my lips and bud. Sometimes he darts his tongue inside, but mostly it stays outside. One of them asks to try something different, wanting to know what will happen if you try to suck on the clitoris. The older one allows him to try, cautioning him to be extremely gentle.

217

At one point the older man is holding me open, so that they may all learn the female anatomy and female responses. He begins to stroke me gently. As my juices start to run and I begin to writhe about, he removes the stroking hand, leaving me exposed so that they can watch the results. He doesn't leave me too long in that tortured state, but quickly removes his clothes and begins to gently massage me even more; my breasts, my cunt, my arse. He reminds them not to neglect any sexual or erogenous area of a woman's anatomy.

When it is clear that we are both at the peak of arousal, he enters me and stays in deep, while I go completely mad all around him. He pulls almost all the way out and randomly touches various sensitive parts of my internal anatomy, and the situation goes to automatic pilot. At some time during the beginning of my orgasm, I am barely aware of the young men touching me, sucking on my breasts or caressing my arse while I'm coming. They are still dressed. Naturally, after a period of refreshment, the young men want to try. They are allowed to do so, but the older man stays to offer guidance.

Sophie, 19, Photo Studio Assistant
I fantasise a few times a week. The fantasies depend on my mood and if I'm with my partner. They range from sex with dogs and strangers to muscular men and being blindfolded and restrained. I used to get turned on a lot by porn magazines and lingerie, such as black or white lace underwear. I also still like the idea of doing it outside in public. The idea of being blindfolded, which I have now tried, is very horny, as is being really noisy during sex.

I normally have this fantasy when I'm walking up to my fiancé's house, as the walk is quiet and boring. It starts when my fiancé comes up to me in a pub or club.

218

It is very hot and the place is packed. The more we dance, the hotter it gets and the hotter I get. He starts undoing his top to show his torso and chest and then starts to unzip my dress, which is zipped up the front. Nobody is looking, but it feels as if they are.

Eventually, I turn my back on him. He feels me up from behind, running his hands up and down my stomach and breasts. Then he covers my mouth with one hand and, with the other, he inserts his penis into me. As we dance back and forth, we climax rhythmically to the music. I vary my fantasy slightly, depending on how long my journey takes, and you will never guess what I'm gagging for when he sees me walking up the path!

Monica, 24, Student Nurse

I like to fantasise that I'm starring in a hardcore porno movie, or that I am a high-class escort. It would be a good adventure working late nights, meeting rich businessmen and maybe the odd woman and charging the earth for my services. I also like the idea of being a glamour model. I would love to do a full spread. The idea of all those men jerking off fills me with a feeling of power and pleasure. I would probably wear a nurse's uniform. This must be symptomatic of my desire to be a no-shame, wanton woman. I also like to imagine that I'm in prison with six other women in one cell.

When I was younger, swimming and wearing a bikini were a turn-on. At fourteen, I started buying my own underwear. I always felt good pulling on fresh underwear. Now that I don't wear underwear, it is also a nice turn-on. I like to be on all fours with the man behind me. With women, I enjoy wearing a strap-on dildo, acting out the man's role. Then we swap. I have enjoyed anal sex with another woman, but not with a man yet.

Juliet, 42, Accountant

I enjoy fantasising about quick, anonymous sex in public places, and I often fantasise about sex with a stranger in a meeting or on a train or plane. When I was young I found both male and female homosexuality erotic and I enjoyed blue films, too. One of my most erotic experiences was having sex with a man while several others watched while masturbating. I had a great feeling of control over them.

These days, I like to wear sexy clothing and enjoy letting men glimpse but not touch. I still enjoy both written and visual pornography. I probably like the thought of control in all situations. I also like a man to watch me masturbate. Then I perform oral sex on him, while the man is driving down the motorway. Strange behaviour for a middle-aged, middle-class mother of two!

Lisa, 43, Training Consultant

I fantasise several times a week. They tend to be similar in theme. I'm usually being taken advantage of by some extremely well-endowed male. This is very different from my real-life situation, where I'm usually very much in control. Boring! My breasts, although quite small, are my main source of excitement. My earliest memory is of having a boy's hand up my jumper. It's still a turn-on for me. I recently had a year-long affair with a lovely, lovely man and was very sorry when it ended. We had twelve lovely months together. Sex in every place and position imaginable – except in bed! He was a small man, but he made up for it by being incredibly enthusiastic and innovative. He did things to me that I hadn't even dreamt were possible, and it is a hard act to follow.

My current favourite fantasy goes like this. I meet an old friend. We chat and I discover that I've just moved to the town where he is living. He is married with grown-up children. Later my doorbell rings and his son is on my doorstep. He always had a crush on me in the past, and we chat and have coffee. Suddenly, I notice that he's developed a huge lump in his trousers. He makes his excuses and leaves.

A few days later, he comes back. It is the height of summer and I invite him into the garden for some iced lemonade. He sits down, sips his drink, and I take off my T-shirt to reveal just a very small G-string. Shane doesn't know what to do about the growing bulge in his jeans. I pretend not to have noticed it, and carry on a 'normal' conversation. I make a mess of rubbing oil into my arms, until he offers to help. Then he oils my back, and I turn over and he oils my small breasts. In no time at all, I have stripped him as well.

Later his dad John arrives. He is extremely well endowed and I am still wet and horny from Shane. Soon we are screwing, too. I don't tell one about the other, but we carry on lengthy affairs.

Samantha, 47, Housewife

I like to fantasise often. Some of my favourite themes include watersports, voyeurism, sex in open or public places and sex from behind with a total stranger. I used to get very turned on by black satin or lace garments; ones that showed my body off at its best. I also found a passage in the Bible that I think is extremely erotic. I recommend reading it and taking it seriously; it fires the imagination tremendously. The passage is in *Esther*, chapter 2, verses 8 to 18. The preparation, prior to this woman's marriage and her first sexual act, showed me what it ought to be like and what I would indeed like myself: total relaxation and pampering leading up to the act. *The Perfumed Garden* and the *Kama Sutra* also influenced me to try different things.

I get turned on by most people's points of view

and personal experiences. Reading erotic literature such as Black Lace is always a turn-on. I am excited by the idea of making love in unusual places, such as the garden shed. I like watching erotic films but not meaningless, hardcore porn with endless copulating couples.

My favourite fantasy takes place when I am travelling a long distance through the night and I have to stop at a service station. There I meet a woman. She recommends I get some sleep at her place before I continue my journey. The house is huge. My bedroom has a two-way mirror. I hear and see the woman and her lover having sex. A stranger enters my room and duplicates with me the scene I have been watching. I am taken to new heights and try new things that before I was scared to try. When I am totally satisfied (exhausted, but re-educated), I go on my way again.

At the next service station, I meet a man who recognises my new awakening and takes me home with him. He is tired of women who are passive and unimaginative. He sees in me a potential beyond my wildest imaginings, and he sets about bringing out all my sexuality. It takes time to do this, and I have to stay there several weeks. Each day we try something new. We spend the whole day in sexual pleasure. The rooms in his house are divided up into themes. The bathroom is large, for all sorts of games to be enjoyed. A bath, a shower, a jacuzzi, a toilet, a bidet, a small swimming pool and a fountain all have their pleasurable uses. The dungeon room contains bondage furniture and accessories. Sexual themes continue throughout the house, from the purpose-made kitchen to the conservatories. There is no work to be done, except to give and receive pleasure. Everything else is taken care of by servants. Sometimes others join in or watch.

Eileen, Age unknown, Student
I like the idea of sex in a public place or domination scenarios. When I was fourteen, I read *Web of Desire* and it was superb. I loved the thought of being tied up and being completely at another's mercy. Most of all I loved the power I could have over others: tying them up, their pleasure totally in my hands. My fantasies are more mature and wild now.

My favourite fantasy is very much like one I read in *Web of Desire*. I'm in the lift at work, in a shopping centre. It is a glass lift. It is late at night and I'm going back to work for some papers. In the lift is Jim, the centre's security guard. He is fixing the controls. I get in and press the button to go to the bottom floor. Jim has been working hard and there is sweat running off his well-tanned and muscled chest. His shirt is open. The lift stops slightly above the food hall. The lift jolts and I fall against him. We can't help ourselves and begin to make mad, passionate love on the floor of the lift, with the cleaners and security cameras watching.

Anita, 24, Care Assistant
I like to fantasise about having sex with lots of people around. They are unaware, however, of what's going on. My favourite current fantasy is set in my local nightclub. I am wearing a long but full skirt with nothing underneath. A group of men take bets on who is going to get laid first. The bet is that they will get more money for doing it in the club and even more if they do it within sight of the others.

They look for the girls in the shortest skirts, thinking they will be easy. One of them, however, has noticed my skirt flying up and revealing what's underneath. After a few dances, we sit down. I sit on his knee and feel that he has a hard-on. I'm feeling very horny, because I have never been knickerless before. I undo his trousers and get his cock out. I spread my skirt

223

around and sit on his cock. All his friends are there. He is the first one to pull, but not the last because I work my way round them all.

Shelley, 25, Medical Technical Officer
I have recurring themes in my fantasies of seducing someone at work or of being seduced myself by another woman. I also like the idea of talking dirty on the phone. When I was younger I enjoyed the most obvious sexual signals. I would fantasise about the naked, well-developed male torso or of being with another woman. I also enjoyed the look that told me that I was desired by another. These days, similarly, a gaze held for slightly too long is a turn-on, as is vigorous dancing in the dark with strobe lights. I enjoy going out in sexy underwear and hold-ups, then letting my boyfriend discover the hold-ups.

My current favourite fantasy is slightly hazy. The opening scene is set at work. A wonderful specimen of manhood comes into the department, needing a heart test. I take him into the room and ask him to strip to his waist. A wonderfully muscled torso is revealed and I start to become excited and aroused. He lies on the couch and I apply the patches and wires. As I am taking his reading, I notice his heart rate increasing. I look over to find him watching me with warm brown eyes. Those eyes wander over my body and I start noticing his body. Warm brown skin, large hands, long muscular legs. I notice a bulge in his trousers and look quickly away back to the reading. It is enough to know what he is thinking, and that my mind echoes what he wants.

Sheila, 20, Nursery Nurse
I like fantasising about a variety of sexual situations, such as having sex in public places, being tied up and helpless, rough sex and using sex toys with my partners. I like to watch gay men having sex and get very

224

horny at the thought of being with more than one man at a time, but always with my boyfriend involved. Oiled, well-toned bodies and G-string underwear is a favourite. I particularly like older men who can see the woman inside and not just on the outside. These days I get turned on by the way my boyfriend treats me. He always thinks of me, rather than being selfish. We try lots of new positions and have sex outdoors where anyone could turn up. I get aroused by my boyfriend talking dirty, telling me what he wants to do to me. I also enjoy him masturbating in front of me.

My favourite fantasy is when I am getting ready to go out. I put on sheer, black lace hold-up stockings, a black G-string and black bra. Over the top, I wear a plain, black dress, nothing fancy. My partner sees what I'm wearing and gets turned on. We go out, and all night I tell him what I want to do to him, teasing him and getting him excited. When we walk back home, he says he is dying for the toilet and needs to go down an alley to relieve himself. I go with him. I walk behind him and hold his dick as he urinates. He turns to face me and I bend down and take him in my mouth. I give him a blow job until we hear someone coming. I stand up and kiss him with his penis pressing against my belly. He is still bare, with me covering him up. The people walk past us, not realising he is bare. He then turns me around and pushes me to the wall. He pulls up my dress and pulls my G-string to one side. He plays with me, then enters me from behind and is very rough. When he comes, we go back home and have sex again. This time it is gentle and loving. All the time, he tells me what he wants to do to me and he talks dirty.

Tara, 26, Single Mother
I fantasise often and at the moment my fantasies centre around an Asian guy I fancy. I know that nothing will ever happen and I think that is why I fantasise so much

and with so many different themes. I was sixteen when I lost my virginity. At the time I was going to a bikers club because I was into the music. All those leather jackets and guys with long, flowing hair drove me crazy. I was very promiscuous at that age and had lots of sex in daring places. The fact that we might get caught was a wonderful turn-on.

I still adore men in leathers who have long hair. The smell of petrol and Brut aftershave turns me on. I also love men with those big, come-to-bed eyes. The biggest turn on for me is having someone who is passionately into me and really shows it. My favourite fantasy involves my landlord's son and, even though we have flirted, I know it won't go any further. The scene goes like this: one day he comes round to collect the rent and I am wet with thoughts of him. We do our usual bit of flirting, but this time it changes and he is pinning me down and his hands are all over my body. He keeps telling me how much he wants to fuck me, while his fingers plunge in and out of my wetness. I am on such a high and can't believe my luck. I come, even before I have his gorgeous dick inside me. Then, suddenly, he is fucking me so hard, I'm nearly screaming in pain and pleasure. I don't want this to end. All the time he is telling me what a lovely body I have and how much I turn him on.

Jade, 20, Sales Assistant
Most of my fantasies are to do with my fiancé. Things that we have done together and, of course, things that we have yet to explore. I used to look at my brother's porn magazines and videos. They used to turn me on, but I didn't masturbate until I was about sixteen. I feel more at ease with my body these days, although I'm still conscious of my breasts, which are very large. My fiancé turns me on like no other. I've never had so many orgasms; it's great! Once, he tied me up. That

was a major turn-on for both of us. I suppose my favourite fantasy involves being confident, being strong, and overpowering my fiancé. He and his friends seem to find fantasies a favourite topic of conversation, however! My fantasy would leave them speechless for once.

Here we go. We often all meet at our local club on a Sunday afternoon after my partner, Bruce, has played football. I decide to give them all some extra time and arrange to have a private show in the back room, where I am the centre of attention. There are rows of chairs laid out in front of the stage and gradually each one is filled with all of Bruce's friends. Some slow, sensual music begins to play and I slowly walk on to the stage, wearing tight, black leather trousers and a tight, black crop-top that makes my breasts look even bigger. Bruce's face is an absolute picture as I start to move around the stage, slowly, sensually and erotically rubbing my hands over my breasts. My nipples stand hard and erect. I look into his eyes with such confidence as I slowly step off the stage and walk towards him. I sit astride him and kiss him passionately. I can feel him hardening already. I stand up and walk around all the other lads, rubbing my body against some, kissing others on the cheek and pushing my breasts into the faces of others. As I walk back to the stage, I start to take my top off to reveal a red, lacy basque. I start to undo my leather jeans, pulling them down over my arse, slowly and seductively. Once they are off, all I have left on is my red basque and red stockings.

I continue to dance slowly around the stage in my own little world. I am rubbing my hands over my breasts and in between my legs. Bruce and his mates have stunned faces and I can see their erections forming in their trousers. I walk forward and kneel in front of Bruce. I rub my hands up the insides of his thighs until my hands meet at his crotch. I look up at him with a grin on my face as I start to undo his jeans. I feel so powerful. Everyone is in suspense, wondering what I'm going to do next. I pull down his jeans to reveal his hard cock ready and waiting. I take it gently in my hands and slowly rub it up and down. I then lean forward and take him deep in my mouth. A groan of pleasure passes his lips as I take him deeper and deeper.

I look around the room and notice that some of the lads have started masturbating. This gives me the courage to carry on, knowing that what I am doing is really turning them on. I then stand up and sit on top of his cock. It fills me deeply and I feel my body heating up as my orgasm approaches. I ride him slowly, grinding myself into him. I look deep into his eyes and he smiles with satisfaction. I start to fuck him faster and he moans in ecstasy as he frees my breasts and sucks on my erect nipples. Our lovemaking becomes extremely intense as we both reach the verge of our orgasms. With one final thrust from him, we both shout out in pleasure and I feel his liquid flow into mine. The other lads are all sitting there with their cocks in their hands, coming all over the place. With a final kiss for my fiancé, I get off him and pick up my clothes and walk back on to the stage and out of the back door.

I didn't realise that this was going to be so long. It just proves what you can do if you put your mind to it. I hope you enjoyed reading this; I know I certainly enjoyed writing it!

Janice, 37, Homemaker
I like reading sexy books on a regular basis and enjoy watching films where the two females make love to each other. I enjoy sharing erotic fantasies with my husband and we often fight over who will read the

Black Lace books first. I fantasise a few times a week and a recurring theme is of being on a stage with a partner. We are making love with an all-male audience, members of which are able to take part if they wish. I used to go and see *Emmanuelle* films with an old boyfriend and particularly remember a massage scene and an acupuncture scene that at the time were a great turn-on.

Chloe, 33, Personal Assistant

I fantasise on average once a day. I have recurring themes such as giving a quick blow job to a stranger in the street or having sex with an audience watching. I also like the idea of sex with several guys at once. I was brought up to be a 'good girl'. However, I have always enjoyed looking at pictures of naked men, especially hairy men. This usually occurred under the bedclothes with a torch, in my teens. Unfortunately, my first husband was of the opinion that wives don't enjoy sex and that licking me out was disgusting.

My second husband has unravelled my head and created a sex monster. I love sex! I love reading about it in explicit detail and watching hardcore porn videos. Watching double penetration has me orgasming in seconds. (I would like to try this one day.) Watching and practising anal sex is a great turn-on. I am now a great exhibitionist and love flashing at strangers. The older I get the hornier I get.

My favourite fantasy is set in a club on Ladies' Night. I have been dragged along by my friend, as I do not really like the handsome stripper look. I prefer the rugged look. A lot of strippers have their chest hair shaved off. The first two strippers are perfectly handsome with not a trace of chest hair in sight. However, the third leaps on to the stage dressed as a fireman. Handsome he is not, but horny he definitely is. My cunt twinges. I can feel myself getting wet as he gyrates fully clothed on stage, wielding an axe above his head. He starts moving around his screaming audience, but I am strangely calm in my arousal. I want him as he starts to strip, throwing his clothes into the audience. Then his top is off and, Oh God, look at the hair on that broad chest! His trousers are off. He has a fantastic body: broad shoulders, slim hips and muscles that are perfectly defined, although he is not muscle bound. He turns around and he even has a fine covering of hair across the back of his shoulders. My cunt takes over. I am soaking wet. He moves back into the audience, ignoring the screaming women, seemingly making a bee-line straight for me. My heart starts to pound. But no, he stops and lets a couple of women rub baby oil down his G-string. I cannot take my eyes off him. He is so horny. Suddenly, he is in front of me, staring me straight in the eyes. He holds out his hand to me and I take it. I feel like I'm in a daze and yet totally in control; I must be dreaming. We walk up to the stage. I'm shaking, although whether through nerves or sexual longing, I'm not quite sure.

He does the usual routine of throwing a flag over my head and upper body, while simultaneously pushing me on to my knees in front of him. The crowd are roaring with approval as he starts bucking into my face, my lipstick smudging against his G-string. His buttocks must look good as they repeatedly thrust into my flag-covered head and upper body. He continues to pretend to fuck my face for a little longer, but the smell of him is finally too much. I've had enough of this simulated oral sex. I want to suck his cock for real. With unusual dexterity I release his cock and with the next thrust he is in my mouth. He pauses momentarily. Does the surprise show on his face? I would love to be able to see his face now. Then the crowd's cheering becomes louder and I know that his brief pause has given the game away. They know that I am sucking his cock underneath that flag. But, my God, he is so thick! I have difficulty getting my mouth around him as he grows in size. I bring my hands up to help my mouth and it is only then that I really appreciate the true stature of this magnificent cock. Not only is it fat, but it is also very long. My cunt floods. I can feel that my knickers are now soaked with my juices. I have always wanted to worship a monster like this. I hear him grunt and his cock twitches. I pull away and just tickle his balls and arsehole very gently. Suddenly the flag is pulled off me and his cock is back behind the G-string. (As much of it as is possible anyway.) The crowd is yelling and roaring its approval as he stands me up to take a bow. I look him straight in the eyes, and it is now his eyes that are glazed with lust.

'On your hands and knees,' he commands. 'Arse to the audience.'

Immediately, I obey. My short, flared miniskirt rides up to reveal my white panties. He drops to his knees behind me and begins to thrust at my rear, his arse clenching and relaxing.

'You bitch,' he rasps in my ear. 'You're wearing stockings.' I turn my head and spit back at him, 'Why don't you just fuck me properly instead of this pretend shit. Go on, fuck me. Now. On stage.'

He reaches for the flag, never interrupting his simulated fucking, and drapes it around our hips. The crowd yells. I feel him fiddling with my panties and finally he loses patience and just rips them aside. His cock is out of its confines again and now I feel it nudging at my opening. All I can hear is the deafening roar of the audience. I risk a glance behind me. Some women are shielding their eyes or have turned away, but the majority of them are on their chairs, screaming and chanting. 'Fuck me, you arsehole!' I hiss at him.

The pause in his rhythm has the women in the audience at fever pitch. Slowly he eases his huge cock into my wet, open and aching cunt. I shout out, throwing my head back. Oh, my God! I cannot take this, surely. I feel like I'm being split in two. He pauses, once he is in me ball deep, to give me a chance to adjust to his size. There is nothing in my world now, apart from the hysterical shouting of the audience and his cock buried deep inside me. The flag is still concealing the true nature of events. He starts to pump. He grabs a handful of my hair and pulls my head back. The flag slips slightly. I hear a guttural growling and realise that it is me. The crowd starts to chant, 'Off, off, off, off, off, off,' until I pull the flag from his grip and it falls to the floor so that our animal sex is exposed to everyone. I shuffle round, pulling him with me, so that we are side-on to the audience and everyone can see his glistening expanse of cock pistoning in and out of my body.

Suddenly I'm coming. The smell of sex, the chanting of the audience and the fucking I am receiving from this monster of a cock has overwhelmed me. I hear myself shouting over my shoulder to the now redfaced stripper to fuck me harder, because I am coming. At these words, his body shudders and, for the first time in my life, I actually feel a jet of spunk hit my cunt walls as he unloads the contents of his balls into me. He is still pumping. I ride my orgasm and start to come again to huge cheers. I finally scream out my orgasm to the assembled throng.

As he finally slumps over me, the compere rushes on stage and throws the flag over us. The house lights go out moments after to leave us in complete darkness. His cock gradually subsides inside me. I can hear huge applause and stamping of feet coming from the darkness, as I am helped off stage to the dressing room to recover.

Eliza, 29, Engineer

I fantasise several times a day. I enjoy imagining sex with strangers or people I've hardly met. Sometimes I dream about having orgasms, but they never really happen. Sex in public places, blokes with massive cocks and masturbating in front of an audience are also big turn-ons. Smell is an erotic stimulant for me: perfume and aftershave and the smell of my own panties, particularly. These days, as well as smells, fat men, pony tails, dancing and Scottish accents all play a part in my sexual fantasies.

One of my main fantasies is about the white slave trade. When I was eighteen, my Saudi Arabian pen-friend came to stay with us. He had his father's permission to offer my parents two million dollars for me. I fell in love with the guy and we got engaged. He took my virginity. It all came undone when he phoned from an Egyptian whorehouse, telling me what the women there would teach me once I was there.

I fantasise about going to Saudi to be with him. In my fantasy he sends me to 'school' in Egypt and I meet all these beautiful whores. They teach me about my body. I begin to feel things I never knew I could experience. They teach me how to pleasure a man, how to keep him close to orgasm and ride him until he is about to faint. They teach me how to lick and suck him to orgasm. With these teachers I become so good at sex that the richest men want to be with me. The greatest thrill is when I have to dance in front of the king. I wear European clothes and the music begins. It is Arabic and my hips and arms begin to move. The men watching begin to ogle me more intensely. When I take my gear off, I am wearing a see-through top and Arabian trousers. They can see my pale skin and my big tits. My pubes show through. I see them lick their lips. The king sweats as he gets more and more aroused. I swerve around the dance floor and forget about the audience.

I become aroused by the movement and I begin to touch myself as part of my act. When I look again, the men have taken their dicks out. They touch themselves, as they are not allowed to touch me. They moan and I moan. All of us have immense pleasure.

In the end the king can't stand it any more and orders me to relieve him. I oblige only too willingly and the whole scene turns into one big orgy. Other women join in and the smell of sweat and love juices clings in the air. I won't want to leave the harem; I like giving pleasure to these men. They are like putty in my hands and up my arse.

Justine, 30, Chiropodist

I fantasise a couple of times a week and tend to have recurring themes playing in my head. One of my favourites is being with another woman or with other women. I have always enjoyed sneaking a look at a woman's breasts or naked body. I also enjoy fantasising about sneaking off for an illicit session with someone I shouldn't be with. I can be aroused by thinking of gay men together, but it isn't something I would particularly like to see in the flesh.

My favourite fantasy is of being in a live sex lesson. The male teacher is trying to explain sex to a group of innocent girls. He asks how many people have seen a cock for real, and then he ends up pulling down his trousers and showing himself to us. The girls ask to have a touch and he goes around showing himself to the class and letting them have a stroke. Soon he is standing with a proud erection.

He moves on to the female sex organs and chooses me to come to the front. He asks if I will remove my top and bra, which of course I do, and he begins to rub and caress my breasts to show how a man turns on a woman. Then he asks if he can remove my skirt and pants. Then he lays me in front of the class and spreads my legs wide and begins to show the female anatomy to everyone, pointing out my clitoris and vaginal lips, etc., which by now are getting very wet. He slides a finger inside me but, as I am lying flat, I cannot see what he is doing. Then he climbs over me and slides his cock inside me and begins to make love to me in front of the class. This turns into a complete orgy, starting with the other girls getting into pairs to explore each other and then the teacher having a go with as many as he can manage.

Kirstie, 32, Credit Controller/Housewife/Mother
I fantasise a few times a week and like to think about myself with another female and my partner, with another male watching our sexual activities. I used to be crazy about men in jeans with lovely bums and white T-shirts and still get aroused by them to this day. Firemen in uniform are a real turn on, too. I love the TV programme *London's Burning*.

My favourite fantasy is when I am stepping out of the shower. I rub on some light oil moisturiser; it smells wonderful. It is such a warm afternoon that I stay naked, not bothered that I have no net curtains. I get a cold bottle of white wine and sit in the garden, feeling the sun warming my body. I run my hand through my silky pubic hair. I am so warm and starting to feel aroused. My partner, Neil, comes home and, while he showers, I lay myself out on the garden table and wait. Neil comes down to my open legs and feels how wet I am and he makes me wait. He knows that I think about having photos of me in erotic poses and that it really turns me on. The camera clicks away as I perform until I can wait no more. I have to orgasm, oooh . . .

Patricia, 46, Plant Maintainer/Jeweller
I fantasise several times a day and enjoy the idea of being loved and cherished. It must be a savage love

that allows no room for inhibitions at all. I also fantasise about meeting someone, a man or woman, that I just have to make love to. Anywhere, any time. *The Story of O* was one of my first erotic books. Reading about domination is very erotic. Just recently, I watched the film *Damage* and was riveted and turned on by it. I would like to experience a loving, sexual relationship with another woman. I am very turned on by the thought of being able to caress another woman's body, but so far it hasn't happened, and I don't know how to go about it. However, the mind is very powerful and I have very nimble fingers.

My favourite fantasy takes place on a train. It is going to be a long journey. I am devouring my favourite Black Lace book and am so lost in it that I haven't noticed that I'm being watched very closely by the man at the other end of the compartment. We are travelling at night and I'm getting more and more aroused by my book. Suddenly I realise that the man is speaking to me. He asks me what I'm reading. I show him a really explicit chapter, hardly daring to look him in the eye. When I do look at him, he says that he can do better than that. He has condoms and says, 'What about it?'

He pulls me on to his lap and, boy, what a hard-on! We kiss and kiss, his tongue going everywhere and clothes shoved apart for better contact. Then I am lifted and my legs pulled apart for his fingers to do the walking and feeling. My pants are pulled off me and his face is in my crotch. He is licking me. Oh, it is wonderful and I am coming very fast and furiously. The smell of me being licked is mind-blowing. I have to have him. I need to taste him, too, and I need to feel him filling me up and fucking me. He is using me, making me come alive. There is no time for the rest, alas, as the train is stopping. Damn and blast.

Simone, 21, Care Assistant

I like fantasising about moving to the United States. All the American men desire me because I'm English. I also like to fantasise about making love to a prince and marrying him. Prince Andrew is my favourite. I get aroused by the idea of being forced into making love, but I also enjoy thinking about gentle, sweet love-making. My favourite fantasy is set on my wedding night, making love to my husband. We haven't made love before. It is an idea that excites me but would probably never happen. It is, I think, the thought of the innocence and purity of the lovemaking that we would experience.

Denise, 58, Housewife

I fantasise about once a day and tend to have recurring subjects. One of them is of long-lasting lovemaking. I enjoy having my tits sucked and a man's come being massaged into and around my nipples. I get very turned on wanking my friends off. I love them shooting come on to my thick hairy patch, massaging it into my hairs, then replacing my knickers and off I go back to work. What a wonderful lunch break! This used to happen regularly in my teens and early twenties. I love well-developed men in the crotch area! I like to play around with my husband or his friends, sizing up their equipment. I enjoy sucking their tools and then receiving, unannounced, a mouthful of freshly prepared cream.

My current favourite fantasy is of having a large, wide and long tool thrust into my hairy love hole. I am screaming with passionate pleasure as the big boy repeatedly blasts me. At the same time, a second guy is on standby, sucking my tits. When big Rambo number one has filled my love nest with gallons of sperm, number two can jump on and continue the blasting. As number two blasts away, I suck number one back to strength. It is wonderful. I really enjoy my cocktail mixes. I feel I could take at least four full deliveries into the nest, before a short intermission.

Deirdre, 21, Packer

I fantasise several times a day. Books and films were always a turn-on, as were friends telling me about the sex they were having. I like to look at men and wonder what they would be like in bed. One of my strongest fantasies is of wanting a person I know, whom I can't have.

My favourite fantasy of the moment is set at a party where no one knows me. I am wearing very little and all my tattoos are showing. I am drinking and dancing. I get to know a group of people and I go to a hotel and have oral sex with all the women. The men are watching and then they join in. We have loads of sex and drink, and they pay a lot of attention to me, keeping me satisfied. Then it all fades away.

Molly, 26, Mother

I fantasise a couple of times a week. Most involve my husband and I. I used to enjoy dressing up in my mother's stockings and underwear. Even now I find the thought of wearing sexy or kinky clothing a turn-on. Unfortunately, my husband prefers nothing more than baby oil and a smile, so I haven't managed to try this out, yet. I have many different fantasies, ranging from dressing up and being used as a sex object, to using others and exhibiting myself.

Here are some of my most common thoughts. An unknown male knocks at the door. He wants to come in and shows me his business card. We start talking. I am sitting on the edge of the couch. Luckily for him I am wearing a very short skirt and no knickers. He drops something on the floor, right in front of me. I see him try to get a better view under my skirt. I open my legs a bit more. I notice his eyes open wide as I expose my fanny to him. I keep my pubes very short, so nothing spoils his view. I am starting to feel very turned on at this point and can feel my cunt becoming moist. He must notice this, as he says he likes what he sees. I lie back on the couch, lifting my skirt as I do. I cannot see what he does next, but I can feel the warmth of his breath creeping up my thighs. He starts sucking at my cunt and probing me with his tongue. It isn't long before I come all over his face. He wipes himself clean, makes his excuses and leaves.

Sandy, 29, Career Woman
I fantasise several times a week. I tend to think about my boyfriend making love to me. I have always enjoyed sex. Magazines and books were my first intro- duction to it. Most experiences were a turn-on and I had tried most things in my late teens, but never involving children or animals, of course. These days, I like telling my boyfriend dirty stories in bed.

My biggest fantasy is with my boyfriend. I am dressed in black underwear, stockings and G-string, etc. I am bent over the bonnet of a car and he is making love to me from behind. It is night-time and raining hard. I can feel the hard rain while he is pounding me. I am also wearing stilettos and my hair is down. My other fantasy is set in a room on a table. I am on my back with a teacher standing by me. He is using me as a subject in a sex class.

Susannah, 25, Team Manager
I enjoy flirtation in the office and like thinking about what other women or men would be like. I like watch- ing suggestive films but not blue movies. I also enjoy smutty, one-to-one conversations; realising that the other party is being aroused by the conversation is a real turn-on. Board games with a twist can be arousing also. A recurring theme in my fantasies is of two men and myself in a large bathroom with a sunken bath, or

two women and myself on stage, following on from an erotic dance routine.

My favourite fantasy is of being asked to fill in for a girl in a dancing group, on a bar-top stage. I am dressed only in flimsy and sexy underwear and am losing myself in the tempo of the music. I join a tall, long-legged, black beauty on a chaise longue above a circle of gawping men. We start to run our mouths and tongues over each other's bodies. We are both becoming more and more aroused. After exhausting the tantalising effect of mouths around black and white hard nipples, we both move so that our cunts are exposed to each other's mouths and the men's excited stares. We start to lap at each other, penetrating each other's holes with manicured nails. After bringing each other to an amazing orgasm, we select four gentlemen from the audience and tie them in a circle by their wrists. We tease and suck them in turn, until, just prior to their climax, we tire of their bodies and return to the sweet flesh of the other woman. We watch our victims lose total control over their members.

Liza, 18, Unemployed
I like to fantasise a couple of times a month. When I was first discovering my sexuality, I went through a phase of staring at women's breasts in tight tops. I still like clothes as a turn-on: little, short dresses, and long, transparent dresses. In general I like clothes that look sexy but not sleazy. Older men are also a turn-on for me.

My favourite fantasy comes from a book. It involves being a stripper with a lovely body. Each night I'm performing, I get to choose a man to come up on stage with me and do whatever I say to please me. Once we have had some fun, he takes me from behind in front of everybody. I just throw him away when I am finished.

Sylvia, 24, Machine Operator

I fantasise several times a day and a lot of my fantasies tend to take place in enclosed spaces, such as storerooms or pressed up against a wall, etc. I find this strange because I don't like small spaces. I used to get turned on by famous pop or film stars and guys at school. I have seen a few soft and hardcore porn films that my friend's dad had. I felt uncomfortable in front of him and my friend. I tried to laugh it off, saying it was disgusting, but despite my words I still found it arousing and I even had fantasies based on what I had seen.

I like leather-clad men with long, dark hair and motorbikes, or the exact opposite: smart men in business suits with ties, etc. I also get very turned on by a particular guy at work who features in my favourite fantasy. I find this guy completely horny. He makes me feel hot whenever he's around at work. Everything he does, even running his fingers through his hair, makes my stomach flip over. If he ever looks at me or comes anywhere near me I get so wet and my legs go so weak, I'm afraid to stand up. He is tall, dark and gorgeous, but also very shy with women so I have no chance. I'm quite shy too. He wears a suit and has a much higher job than me. I like power. I dream of him a lot and know everything I can about him.

My favourite fantasy with him is usually up against a wall or in a storeroom. I go into his office, walk up to him and bend down to lightly kiss his neck. He turns around and asks what I am doing. I reply that I have to have him or I will go crazy. I sit on his lap, facing him and start to kiss him gently, trying to make him respond. At first he is all tensed up, but soon he opens his mouth and I kiss him so deeply I'm practically eating him. He kisses me back just as passionately. I stop and get up; so does he. I pull him along by his tie until we get to a wall. I push him against it and push myself against him. He says, 'No!' and stops me. He then turns me around and pushes me against the wall. He pushes his body hard against mine and starts kissing my neck. He travels up to my face and kisses my lips hard and starts exploring my mouth with his tongue. I get so hot and start breathing heavily and moaning. His hand starts to slide up my leg under my skirt. My hands are on his bum, through his trousers, and entangled in his hair, pushing his mouth harder on to mine. His hand slides up on to my bum and pulls it hard against his trousered dick.

He keeps whispering into my mouth about how much he has always wanted me but was too shy to do anything about it. He keeps telling me what he would like to do to me. Meanwhile both his hands are rubbing themselves up and down my bum and back, into my hair, burning their way into my skin as they go. Suddenly he pulls back and starts undoing my shirt. He takes it off and then takes off my bra. I'm standing there, getting very hot. He touches my bare skin and I gasp. He then looks into my eyes so deeply, and those lovely dark eyes tell me exactly how he feels at that very moment.

I start to pull off his tie and undo his shirt and pull it out of his trousers. I touch his bare chest and we both realise we won't be able to hold back long enough to take all the rest of our clothes off in the same way. So we just push our bodies together. He pulls up my skirt and takes off my knickers with one quick movement. He unzips his trousers and takes out his dick. He lifts up my leg and I bend my knee and place my foot against the wall, so he can get good access, and we start fucking hard. While we kiss deeply, we come together and hold on to each other for a while. We then pull apart and get dressed, kind of shyly. We hardly look at each other. He goes back to his desk and computer and I go out the door and back to work.

Gwen, 21, Student

I fantasise a few times a week. I used to get aroused by certain books: Anais Nin's *Delta of Venus* and *The Pearl*. A film that turned me on was *Goodfellas* – all that money, power and Italian men! Also, *The Blue Lagoon* – being on a deserted desert island is certainly a turn-on. Generally, reading any erotica has always been a big turn-on. My partner at the moment is very sexy, but so too is the memory of my first sexual partner: my boss at work. Certain TV personalities do it for me: Michael French, who played David Wicks in *EastEnders*, and Ross Burden, the TV Chef: a combination of food and sex!

My current favourite fantasy is set in an airport. I am with my boyfriend and we are feeling very horny. We spy a staff only entrance which is made of thick plastic strips. We dart behind them and my boyfriend hoists me up against a wall. I put my feet on two boxes and we start to make love. We realise then that although we couldn't see in through the plastic strips, we can actually see out. As we continue to make love, we can see all the people in the departure lounges. This really turns us on and I orgasm madly, still shoved against the wall.

Selina, 31, Housewife

I love the idea of being made love to where people might see us. The thrill of being caught or arousing somebody else as they watch is very erotic. When I met my husband I was very unworldly when it came to sex. I read about it more than experienced it. I find all types of sex a turn-on, except for certain S&M. My husband doesn't like any type of pain, just pure pleasure. In the early days we experimented with anything and everything from bananas to Mars bars. We also watch porno films, which I find thoroughly exciting. Now I find making love in places where people can catch us a turn-on. My husband using his tongue and a vibrator is very exciting. Although I am not bisexual I love watching women together. Reading sexy books gets me all wet as well.

My fantasy is based on an actual event. It happened on our way home from Paris by bus. My husband and I were sitting near the back. I was feeling cold and tired, so I pulled my husband's coat over me and laid my head on his lap. Opposite us was a businessman. He kept looking over from time to time. As I laid my head down I could feel my husband's cock hardening. I rubbed my cheek up and down over it. I was getting so turned on. My cunt was wet and throbbing. I could feel my husband moving and moaning and he reached down and unzipped his fly. His cock was so warm and smelt wonderful. As I looked over, the businessman had started rubbing his bulge that had appeared. My cunt was throbbing.

I pulled the coat over me and swallowed my husband's cock. I licked and sucked and teased his balls until his warm come flooded my mouth. As I sat up I noticed the man opposite had pulled his briefcase across himself. My cunt was nearly exploding by this time. My husband slipped his hand up my skirt to my wet knickers and then pushed his warm fingers into me. I wanted him to push his whole hand inside me, I was so wound up. It didn't take me long to flood over his fingers. I don't know what happened to the man opposite. I was too busy licking my husband's fingers.

Amy, 49, Author/Publisher
I fantasise a few times a week and each fantasy tends to be very different. However, I like imagining I have joined the mile high club or am making love in lavishly rich or romantic places. I also enjoy fantasising that I am in semi-private public places, where no one realises

or is aware of our presence. I've always loved and enjoyed fulfilling sex and my lover is a big turn-on. To be truthful, I only enjoy fantasies I can make come true, otherwise there's no point. I enjoy making love in lots of different places. One of my two favourites was a Christmas lunch on the Orient Express. It was only a quickie in the loo, but none the less memorable. The other was in a lay-by off a junction on the M25, one summer evening. My boyfriend and I jumped in the back of his car and began a heated lovemaking session and had full, wonderful sex, including oral. Cars were driving past all the time, but we were too heavily engaged in our sex. Our thanks and relief was that no one disturbed us!

Suzette, 20, Receptionist
I like to fantasise at least once a day. The fantasy usually revolves around having sex with my partner in different settings or positions. My favourite fantasy is when we are in the Peak District at Grandma's house. We do it behind the sofa while my grandparents are sitting on it. Then we go up to the moors where we do it like rabbits in most positions. I also like the idea of my partner raping me.

Abby, 36, Fashion Consultant
I like to fantasise about having multiple male partners and I also like to imagine myself in a submissive position. I was very naive when I was younger; very unadventurous. I was reluctant to give or receive oral sex. I liked romantic scenarios. Black Lace books were too hot for me! When I met my husband, my education started. Sex in public places was my first real fantasy. These days the idea of unexpected partners or using sex aids is a turn-on. I like taking risks and having sex in public places.

My favourite fantasy is set on my birthday. My husband tells me he has arranged something special. A parcel arrives at lunch time. It contains only sex aids. He gets home and orders me to strip. He blindfolds me and attaches wrist and ankle chains to my nipple rings. I hear men arriving but do not recognise all their voices. The ones I recognise are close friends. I'm horrified but really turned on. We eat dinner. I am fed mouthfuls by different men. Then I am tied in a starburst fashion. I hear noises but no one touches me. Then I feel hands exploring. I can now tell the difference between them. Not one is my husband. I hear his voice: he tells me he is videoing everything. I am subjected to a wonderful session of multiple sex. Oral, vaginal and anal – never knowing who is doing what. I hear the box of sex toys being opened and I am played with for what seems like hours. I am never quite allowed to come. My bonds are released and I am positioned so I can take three men at once. The men leave without me seeing any of them.

Serena, 19, Student
I like to fantasise several times a day. I have a tendency to fantasise about deeply penetrative, passionate and occasionally frantic sex with someone I like at the time. I used to get very horny imagining women in tight-fitting teddies, having sex with each other and several men. Orgies, voyeurism, group sex and lesbianism were and still are a turn-on. Deep, rough and frantic sex from behind and female dominance are very arousing thoughts. I also enjoyed Nancy Friday's *Women on Top*. I once had a leather suit and I used to enjoy the feel of the leather against my naked skin. It enhanced the experience for me. Every time I think about the experience I smile.

I have a number of fantasies that I enjoy when I masturbate. One of the current ones involves voyeurism. I am on holiday somewhere exotic and I'm too hot in bed one night. I get up and go down to the pool for a quick skinny-dip to cool myself down, but when I get there, I hear something. I stop dead to try to find out where the noise is coming from. Quietly I slip over to the door leading out to the pool and I find that a couple has beaten me to it. A young woman is naked and lying along the edge of the pool. She sits up to speak to a young man. I'm afraid he will see me so I hide behind a large plant. The young man grabs the woman and spreads her legs. He begins to finger her and she groans with pleasure. He slowly licks his way down to her clitoris and she opens her legs wider. She pushes her vagina against his face and he delves his tongue deep inside her. She moans again and rocks rhythmically against his mouth as she rubs her clitoris and he fingers her vagina and anus.

Linda, 24, Housewife

I fantasise several times a day. The recurring ones tend to be about being picked up in a bar by another woman who is a complete stranger. She pays me to have sex with her. I have always found people's eyes very sexy; eyes that show no emotion. I also still get turned on by music by Enigma. It takes me to a different time and place where I can be anyone and do anything. These days I get turned on by people who have a dangerous edge to them; someone whom I cannot read – that is why I like unreadable eyes. I also like sexy, soft voices. But what turns me on the most is when my husband runs his fingers over the back of my thighs. It makes me so horny.

My favourite fantasy is that I am sitting in a local café, waiting for my sister. I am sitting there drinking a Coke and smoking a cigarette. The café is packed, when a tall man with shoulder-length hair and amazing blue eyes walks in. He asks me if he can join me and if I am waiting for someone. When I tell him I am waiting for my sister, he smiles. He says he is in town for business. While he is talking to me, he is staring. His eyes are unreadable. I offer to show him the way to the museum.

We walk through the town, down behind the city walls to the museum. He asks if I would like to join him. I agree and we walk in. As we enter he pulls me into a corner. He pulls me close and turns me around, so I am facing away from him. He runs his hands over my thighs and over my bum. He lifts up my skirt and runs his hands over the front of my pants. He pulls them down and feels that I am wet and then enters me from behind. He moves very slowly and brings me to orgasm. Just as I am climaxing, someone walks by. We leave quickly and say goodbye.

Eleanor, 17, Student
I like fantasising about seducing close friends or work-mates and being totally dominated. I used to get very horny thinking about men in uniform or tuxedos. These days, sex in public places is a turn-on, as are men working out in the gym.

My favourite fantasy takes place in the warehouse at work. I am walking around with the store manger and we are getting very agitated because we can't find anywhere to be alone together. When everyone finally goes home we start to kiss passionately. His hands are all over me and he slowly strips my clothes off and starts caressing my body. Then I start to take his suit off and I run my hands all over his body. He kisses every square inch of my body and then he lays me out on his desk and starts to fondle me. I try to do the same, but he won't let me. I am completely under his control. He then proceeds to make passionate love to me. We walk out of the office together and go to the customer service desk. He gives me a kiss before we both go our separate ways.

Jocasta, 21, Care Assistant

I fantasise several times a day and like the idea of being in busy, public places, such as country parks, or having sex with someone spying on us. Before I met my current boyfriend, I had never experienced a climax, so I was very naive and thought sex was just for men. I get very turned on by just being with my boyfriend. Every time we have sex, it is a different and wonderful experience for me and he takes great pride in my orgasms as he knows they are a new great experience.

I have a lot of fantasies that I want to try out. One of them is to go abroad and meet a man who is totally shy and sweet. Here goes: I meet him in a bar and I do the chatting up, as he is so shy. I ask him, Jamie, to walk me back to my apartment. The beach is secluded and dark and feels great under bare feet. I feel the waves lap on to my feet and I try to get Jamie to walk with me closer to the sea. I hear him swallow. I know he wants me but is too shy to do anything about it. So I decide I have to do all the work. I start to unbutton my own shirt, feeling the sea breeze on my hardening nipples. I see Jamie looking. I pull him close to me and he eventually bends down to kiss me. His tongue is at first as shy as his personality, then it gets more probing and eager. I feel Jamie's hand on my bare breasts. At first he uses small, gentle strokes but as his tongue probes more into my mouth the strokes turn to eager grasps and pinches that are so delightful. I push myself towards Jamie's groin and I know that his penis is hard and eager, so I unbutton his jeans. This is when I see him for the first time. He is so thick and strong, the head of his penis jerking to my every touch. Jamie's mouth opens and he makes a quiet whimpering noise. I am dying to feel his thick manhood inside me, but I want to make him beg me for some sort of release.

I pull Jamie further into the water and I feel the

coldness of the salty water on my pubic hair. I can feel my excitement rising even more. We grab each other and kiss so urgently that it nearly hurts. Jamie lifts up my skirt and puts his long fingers on my clitoris, which is so hard and longing for any caress. He at first moves his finger painfully slowly, but then he gets faster. I feel a warmth in my stomach and I know my release is near. I reach for Jamie's penis and start to masturbate him vigorously. I hear moans and I'm not sure whose mouth they are coming from. Jamie's fingers move faster and he slips one into my wet vagina. I feel his fingers moving and I feel my orgasm coming. I know that only a few more strokes will send me into an hysterical mess. I feel Jamie's penis getting even thicker and I can hear the air trapping in his throat and I know that Jamie is close too. I start to masturbate him even harder until I hear him moan and jerk and then I see his milky seed hurling into the sea. Seeing Jamie's excitement unlocks the trapped orgasm from inside me. I feel wave after wave of warm fluttering. We kiss gently, gather our wet, sandy clothes and dress in utter silence. Then we walk our separate ways up the dark, quiet beach away from each other.

Valerie, 38, Housewife/Mature Student
I fantasise a couple of times a week and I tend to have fantasies that suggest overcoming inexperience. I have only slept with one man and my other experiences were basic fumblings. The first time I got interested in fantasising was when I saw an *Emmanuelle* movie. I started to wonder what it would be like to be her. My only sexual experience at the moment is watching videos or reading erotica. The sex I have now is with myself and a vibrator.

One of my favourite fantasies takes place in the 1920s. A young innocent girl goes to live with distant relatives. There she is brought to life sexually by both her distant cousins and their staff. She is shown how to pleasure herself and how to give and receive pleasure from another woman. Even the boot boy helps to educate her. Soon everybody is giving and receiving pleasure from each other.

Another fantasy is of a young girl who goes to work at a hotel. There she learns more about life from staff and visitors alike. On her first day she is told to change the linen on one floor. She is told to knock and wait for an answer. If there is no answer she is to go in with her pass key. She comes to the last door. She knocks and waits, but gets no reply, so she goes in. What she sees stops her in her tracks. A beautiful woman is lying naked on the bed. She is writhing with pleasure because she is using a vibrator that fits into both her vagina and her anus, sending shivers of pleasure through her body. The young girl makes a slight sound and the woman smiles. The girl makes a quick exit but she finds that her panties are damp and she is feeling something she doesn't understand. She meets the woman again and gets to experience the pleasure herself. Soon she is having fun with both men and women in the hotel.

My third favourite fantasy is about a mature woman who has only ever slept with one man. (Ring any bells?) She then has a succession of experiences with both men and women in a dress shop, where more than her measurements are taken. She also gets involved with a rather handsome young man when she has her hair cut privately.

Veronica, 28, Secretary
I watch hard-porn videos to get me in the mood; ones with lots of willies and oral sex turn me on. I love fantasising about having sex with two men at once: one fucking me up the bum and the other up the fanny. I also love fantasising about sex with black men

(especially the footballer Ian Wright) or sex with my neighbour in his house and car.

My current favourite fantasy involves meeting up with this guy called D. We go out to the woods in his sports car. We get out in a quiet spot, sit down and begin to kiss. Little kisses at first, then deep probing ones with our tongues. I begin to unbutton his shirt and then pull it off. I kiss his bronzed chest all the way down until I find his belly button which I proceed to stick my tongue into. I then undo his jeans noticing a hard lump in his trousers. His great big hard prick springs free and I take it in my mouth and begin to suck it, licking it up and down, moving my tongue in and out of his hole. He is groaning now and I feel him getting harder. By this time I am naked and very wet. He takes his prick and puts it in my anus and begins to fuck me slow and hard and at the same time he finger fucks my fanny. We both come together. He then gives me a long cuddle and a lingering kiss.

Afterword

*I*t has been a privilege to have had access to such fascinating material during the time it has taken to compile this book. The defining factor of all the fantasies that were submitted to this project is the unbridled enthusiasm for pleasure. We should try to allow as much of it into our lives as we can. As the philosopher Joseph Campbell said, 'It's important to find your bliss.'

Being repressed and shamed by an aspect of human existence which is as old as existence itself is a great nonsense, and should be left behind with the end of this millennium. Repressive censorious dogma makes for ill individuals and societies. Sometimes I think there's a worldwide conspiracy at work. We are attracted to what we're not allowed to have and by what we are told is naughty. We're all pretending to be shocked by unconventional sexuality, but the truth is that we're fascinated. Sexually alluring pictures and salacious stories are used to sell newspapers every day. But what often lies behind sensationalist articles are moral warnings which attempt to brew up guilt or anger about being gay, lesbian, unmarried at thirty, sexually active at fifty, or just different and defiant. Every time we read a reactionary piece of journalism we know we're being cheated and manipulated but we don't want to admit it. It's like the fable of the Emperor's New Clothes: we're all pretending not to be conned.

Perhaps we can change things in a small way. We can start by rejecting sensationalist headlines which whip up hysteria and knee-jerk reactions. Next time someone asks you 'Did you hear about the gay/kinky/adulterous MP?', why not reply, 'Yes, I did, but I think he's been a victim of double standards'? It's time to reject hypocrisy and bring about a new Age of Enlightenment where we can recognise the differences in each other and accept them, and science and technology can work for the good of humankind, and hatred and inequality can be obliterated. Oh well, I've always been an idealist. For now, it's best we enjoy ourselves. At least we live in exciting times!

Kerri Sharp
December 1998

Contacts

UK

Organisations

Feminists against Censorship
Feminists fighting for free expression and diversity for all
BM FAC, London WC1N 3XX
tel: (0181) 552 4405

Libertarian Alliance
Promotes libertarian ideas, including sexual freedom and opposition to censorship
Chapter Chambers
Esterbrook St
London SW1P 4NN
tel: (0171) 821 5502

SM Pride
Straight, gay and bi pervs celebrate SM in a big annual
event with workshops, demonstrations and a big party
PO Box 10937
London N15 6PE
tel: (0181) 598 2542

Shops and distributors

Sh!
Delightful women's sex shop for clothing and accessories – men welcome only as women's guests
43 Coronet St
London N1 6HD
tel: (0171) 613 5458

Naughty Nostalgia
Stock a wide range of magazines and books, including
vintage material
PO Box 23
Whitby
YO21 3YT
tel: (01947) 821655
email: fiona.clewlow@virgin.net

Paradiso
Rubber, PVC, accessories, lingerie, shoes, books and
jewellery
41 Old Compton Street
London W1V 5PN
tel: (0171) 287 2487

Publications

Skin Two – Glossy fetish magazine. Great listings section
Unit 63
Abbey Business Centre
Ingate Place
London SW8 3NS
tel: (0171) 498 5533

Forum – Long-standing, informative UK sex magazine for men, women and couples
Northern & Shell Tower
PO Box 381
City Harbour
London E14 9GL
tel: (0171) 308 5090

Desire Direct – Extensive contact ads magazine, for men, women and couples
Moondance Media Limited
192 Clapham High St
London SW4 7UD
tel: (0171) 627 5155

US

Organisations

Feminists For Free Expression
2525 Times Square Station
New York, NY 10108–2525
tel: (212) 702 6292
freedom@well.com

Society of Janus
Pansexual educational and social group. Newsletter,
parties, discussions
PO Box 426794
San Francisco
CA 941412–6794
tel (415) 985 7117

NLA (National Leather Association International)
Annual Living in Leather conference. NLLA has chapters in many cities. Send a SASE to national head-
quarters for information about local chapters.
584 Castro St, #444
San Francisco
CA 94114–2500

Shops

Good Vibrations – Women's sex shop
1210 Valencia Street
(at 23rd Street)
San Francisco
CA 94110
tel: (415) 974 8980

Toys in Babeland – Women's sex shop
94 Rivington Street
New York NY 10002
tel: (212) 375 1701

or

707 East Pike Street
Seattle WA 98122
tel: (206) 328 2914

Good For Her
181 Harbord Street
Toronto Canada
tel: (416) 588 0900

Cool Websites
http://www.blowfish.com
http://underwire.msn.com
http://www.bust.com
http://www.babeland.com
http://www.a-womans-touch.com
http://www.goodforher.com
http://www.fiawol.demon.co.uk/fac
http://www. well.com/user/freedom

Virgin Publishing Ltd accepts no responsibility for errors or dissatisfaction arising from contact with any of the above.

Notes

Chapter One – A Personal History:
Good Girls, Bad Girls and Why Fantasies Matter
1. John Berger, *Ways of Seeing*, p. 47, BBC/Penguin Books Ltd, London, 1972
2. Ibid., p. 53
3. Lydia Lunch, *Suture*, p. 25 Creation Books, London, 1998
4. Avis Lewallen, 'Lace: Pornography for Women?' *The Female Gaze*, eds. Lorraine Gamman and Margaret Marshment, p. 89, The Women's Press Limited, London, 1988
5. Ibid., p. 101
6. Alison Assiter and Avedon Carol, *Bad Girls and Dirty Pictures*, p. 17, Pluto Press, London, 1993
7. Ibid., p. 16

Chapter Two – Stranger Attractions:
Anonymity Guaranteed
1. Laura Lee Davis and Hallet Arendt, 'Transports of Delight', *Time Out* Magazine, pp. 28–30, December 9–16 1998

Chapter Three – Bountiful Lust:
Puritans and Libertines, The Group-Sex Fantasy

1. St Thomas Aquinas, *Summa Theologica*, questions 92, 35, Eyre & Spottiswoode, New York, London*
2. Karen Armstrong, *The Gospel According to Women: Christianity's Creation of the Sex War in the West*, p. 69, Doubleday, New York, 1986*
3. *Apocrypha*, Ecclesiasticus, 25: 13–26*
4. Rossell Hope Robbins, *The Encyclopaedia of Witchcraft and Demonology*, Bonanza Books, New York, 1981*
5. Jonathan Miller, *The Don Giovanni Book of Myths, Seduction and Betrayal*, Faber & Faber, London 1990

* All quotes sourced from Helen Ellerbe, *The Dark Side of Christian History*, Morningstar Books, 1995

Chapter Four – Gender Play

1. Kenneth MacKinnon, 'Gay's the Word – Or Is It', *Pleasure Principles: Politics, Sexuality and Ethics*, eds, Victoria Harwood, David Oswell, Kay Parkinson and Anna Ward, p. 121, Lawrence & Wishart, London 1993
2. Ibid., pp. 112–113

Chapter Five – The Sexual Submissive

1. Anita Phillips, *A Defence of Masochism*, p. 72, Faber and Faber, London, 1998
2. Ibid., p. 3
3. Ibid., p. 89

The Dark Man of the Psyche

1. Sigmund Freud, *Creative Writers and Day-Dreaming, The Pelican Freud Library*, volume 14: Art and Literature
5. Michelle Olley, 'Once Upon a Time', *Skin Two Magazine*, p. 64, issue 22
8. Ibid.
9. Angela Carter, *Burning Our Boats*, p. 459, Chatto and Windus Limited, Random House Group, London, 1995
10. Clarissa Pinkola Estés, *Women Who Run With the Wolves*, p. 66, Random House Group Limited, London, 1992

Chapter Six – Bondage, Punishment, and All the Trimmings

1. Avis Lewallen 'Lace: Pornography for Women?', *The Female Gaze*, eds. Lorraine Gamman and Margaret Marshment, p. 100, The Women's Press Limited, London, 1988

Chapter Seven – Not Just Bodies
Kinky Boots, Leather Lovers, Punks and Nazis

1. Susan Sontag, 'Fascinating Fascism', *Under the Sign of Saturn*, p. 99, Farrar Stratus Giroux, 1972
2. Ibid., p. 105
3. Dick Hebdidge, *Subculture, The Meaning of Style*, pp. 107–108, Routledge, London, 1993

Chapter Eight: Loving Ourselves to Bits

1. Nancy Friday, *Women on Top*, p. 9, BCA, London, New York, 1991

Bibliography

Bataille, G, *Eroticism*, Marion Boyars, London, 1987

Cope, J, *The Modern Antiquarian*, Thorsons, Harper-Collins, London, 1998

Cowan, L, *Masochism – A Jungian View*, Spring Publications, Inc., Dallas, 1992

Ellerbe, H, *The Dark Side of Christian History*, Morningstar Books, 1995

Friday, N, *Women on Top*, BCA, London, New York, 1991

Miller, J, ed., *The Don Giovanni Book of Myths, Seduction and Betrayal*, Faber & Faber, London, 1990

Phillips, A, *A Defence of Masochism*, Faber & Faber, London, 1998

Sjöö, M, and Mor, B, *The Great Cosmic Mother*, Harper, San Francisco, 1987

Steele, V, *Fetish Fashion, Sex and Power*, Oxford University Press, New York, 1996

Strossen, N, *Defending Pornography: Free Speech, Sex, and the Fight for Women's Rights*, Abacus/Simon and Schuster Inc., New York, 1995